RECLA

Rebel

Here's to having
unconditional love
for your body!
Love,
Lizzy :)

To download your free companion journal pages, scan the QR Code below, or go to www.nutritionbylizzy.com/journal.

Lizzy Cangro
lizzy@nutritionbylizzy.com

ISBN: 978-1-7376315-0-7 (print)
ISBN: 978-1-7376315-1-4 (ebook)

Ordering Information:
Special discounts are available on quantity purchases by corporations, associations, and others. For details, contact lizzy@nutritionbylizzy.com

12 REBELLIOUS ACTS TO ACHIEVE
UNCONDITIONAL LOVE FOR YOUR BODY

RECLAIM THE
Rebel

LIZZY CANGRO MA, MSc, PGCE, ANutr

To my body,
I love you unconditionally

CONTENTS

READ BEFORE *you* REBEL

Rebels are not wallflowers that settle for second best.

It's Sunday night, and you're lying in bed fretting about tomorrow's to-do list. However, you can barely hear yourself think over the rumbling of your stomach. After a week of your juice cleanse, all you want is to demolish a pizza. In the blink of an eye, reality smacks you in the face—it's now Monday morning, you're hitting the fifth snooze button in a row and making a mad dash out of the house, skipping breakfast, and grabbing a coffee from the local store. On your way into work, you trip in your heels, spraying coffee everywhere—including all over that cute guy from accounting's white shirt. Blushing, you apologise profusely about how stupid you are and race upstairs.

Sound familiar?

Well, girl, you're not alone. So many of us have developed destructive thoughts and harmful behaviours towards our bodies, such as negative self-talk, being constantly on the go, and cycling through fad diets. This is costing us our mental and physical health, damaging our relationships, and robbing us of our money, time, and energy.

But wait! What if it didn't have to be like that?

Imagine: what would it be like having unconditional love for your body?

You probably spent a nanosecond thinking about that question, didn't you? It's time to sit back down. Do not pass go, and do not collect $200 until you have parked your butt and really thought about it. The fact that you are here shows you want to reclaim unconditional love for your body. If this is really the case, you will make time for this one question:

What does unconditional love for your body look like to you? Go on—be rebellious and dream into this.

I want you to be bold and leave any limitations at the door. Rebels are not wallflowers that settle for second best. The problem comes when we try to be 'realistic'. For example: 'I know I'm not meant to be a runner, so I'll settle for doing a 5k next year at a slow jog'. Or, 'I am beyond busy running my business, so I'll settle for five hours of sleep'. No, No, NO! Settling is not okay. Yes, approach your health and wellness in a sustainable manner, but this doesn't mean setting limitations for yourself.

When it comes to your goals for your health and wellness, there really are no limits. Your vision may be that 'I'll have a spa day every week where I take time for myself and my body'. Or, 'I will be confident on camera and do daily live videos for my business'. I know this is hefty for a lot of women, but I want you to start thinking from a place of possibility, not resignation.

Despite chronically abusing it from a young age, I learnt how to love my body unconditionally. As a 14-year-old, I was severely underweight at 86 pounds, had a pulse of 30 bpm, and was told I was going to die of a heart attack. I am now the international expert in rebellious self love. In this book, I share my most vulnerable experiences with you with the hope of inspiring you to make radical changes in your life for the better.

Anything is possible given the right tools, which you'll acquire in the 12 chapters of this book. These tools take the form of 12 rebellious acts ('RAs') that have transformed my own health and wellness, as well as those of my clients. Following these rebellious acts will lead you to inner peace, joy, and freedom, as well as show you how to confidently step into the body you love.

Are you ready to have some fun as you outrageously craft your dream life without rules?

It's time to rebel.

LIVE YOUR *life* BACKWARDS

Would you continue with the limiting belief of 'I am not enough' if you fully accepted that it robs you of what you want?

What keeps so many of us stuck in life is the feeling that if we only had something, we would then be happy, beautiful, or whatever. When in fact, the key to getting what we want in life is embodying the character traits of the version of ourselves who already has what we want. You need to prioritise the type of person you are before you can obtain your goals. This is living your life backwards.

The Illusion

After graduating with an MSc in nutrition from King's College London, I became an accredited nutritionist with the Association for Nutrition and set up my own private practice. I specialise in helping clients achieve long-term health and wellness using a combination of nutrition, movement, and mindset, which has seen me work with groups and individuals in both the U.K. and U.S.

Some common goals I hear in my practice include 'I want to lose 10 pounds', 'I want a flat stomach', and 'I want better skin'. When I ask my clients why they have these goals, I often hear the following: 'I want to feel better', 'I want to look good', and 'I want to have more energy'.

If we were to dig deeper, these reasons stem from the core belief that 'I am not enough. When I achieve my goal, I will be enough'. A lot of us have some version of this belief.

I blame marketing and consumerism for this.

Think about it. Companies persuade us to buy into their brand by convincing us that we are lacking something, and guess what—they can provide that something through their product! Thank goodness!

In buying into this illusion, we trade away our money, power, and inner peace. Worse, it perpetuates the limiting belief that 'I am not enough', and we need to have something else to be happy and fulfilled.

By holding on to this limiting belief, what we are really saying is that we don't love ourselves. This way of thinking often culminates in multiple failed attempts at long-term health and wellness, frustration, and ultimately, the feeling of being stuck in the same place with the same lack of results.

Would you continue with the limiting belief of 'I am not enough' if you fully accepted that it robs you of what you want?

You're probably now thinking, 'No, Lizzy, of course not!' But so many of us are holding on to this belief.

Our limiting belief of 'not enough' tends to come with a secondary benefit. It may not seem obvious. After all, why would we want to feel 'not enough'? However, this hidden reward is super powerful at keeping us in the same patterns. For example, if I believe I am not a good enough nutritionist and wellness coach, I don't take risks to expand my business or help more people. I therefore avoid having to be vulnerable, I don't have to spend time and money on projects, and life stays predictable (read: safe).

When you are aware of this limiting belief but still attach to it, what you're really saying is that it's more important for you to keep your attachment to not feeling enough and playing things safe than it is for you to achieve your health and wellness goals. Again, you are not practicing self-love.

Now, I'll ask again: how much of this limiting belief are you willing to let go of?

After breaking down in tears on what was supposed to be one of the happiest days of my life, it was a no-brainer for me. I wanted the belief that I wasn't good enough gone.

I was 21 years old and at the end of my undergraduate degree. Three years of a rigorous education were about to be cemented in the grade released. Most students get a 2:1, but I craved getting the top grade: a 'first'. As a perfectionist, I wanted this accolade badly and had sacrificed all my relationships, time, and energy to get it. I hadn't slept or eaten properly in months and had studied every day until my head hurt. My professors expected me to do well, and I'd been offered a post-graduate teaching job because of my stunning predicted grades.

My parents couldn't wait to celebrate the result of my hard work and had driven to Cambridge to walk down to Senate House with me, where exam results are posted in the most public and old-school way possible.

Walking down the avenue into the town centre, I could feel my stomach constricting. Out of the corner of my eye, I could see my dad's knuckles turning white from my squeezing his hand. 'Please be a first. Please be a first', my heart pleaded.

I unclamped my hand and shuffled over to the boards where the results had been posted, trying to get close enough to see my name without having to fight off the gaggle of other nervous finalists from my class. I inched closer to notice the lists were arranged by grade.

'Okay, let's start at the top'.

'FIRSTS'

'No, not me. No, not me. No, no—'

'SHIT'.

Hurriedly checking the 2:1s, I spotted my name.

'Crap'.

I turned my back to the boards and trudged back to my parents. I looked up briefly, finding my dad's eyes glowing with excitement. I burst into tears.

I could feel the warmth of my mum's arms wrap around me. As they both proclaimed how proud they were of me, I inhaled deep breaths of my mum's perfume between sobs and tried to explain how much of a failure I was and why I was crushed.

And then it hit me like a 2x4 to the head. I had so much going for me: I had amazing parents, amazing grades, and an amazing teaching opportunity ahead of me, but all I could see was that 2:1 staring back and telling me I wasn't good enough. A part of me knew in this moment that it was time to give up this limiting belief.

At what point will you decide to give it up too?

The thing is, you were born enough. You are enough now. What's different between now and then is that your brain has been programmed to believe you are not enough. And what's different between you and the people who have what you want in life is that they don't have this limiting belief.

The Rebellious Act

So, what do you have to do, see, or hear to eliminate this limiting belief for yourself? This is the million-dollar question. Well, the problem here is that you are currently living your life out of order, trying to have the outcomes you want without embodying the characteristics of the version of yourself who has those outcomes.

To have what we want in life, whether that's losing 10 pounds, a flatter tummy, or $100,000 in our bank account, we need to embody the traits of the version of ourselves who already has what we want.

Take, for example, my client, Stacy. Stacy, a mum of two kids, desperately wanted to regain her pre-pregnancy body and feel sexy again. She was doing all the right things—working out, eating well, and staying hydrated—but just couldn't ever seem to get to her goal. That was, until she started living her life backwards. She let go of her old identity and reinvented herself in her own mind as a woman who has a great body and the confidence to go with it.

How you 'see' yourself (i.e. your identity), regardless of what is true or not true, is what you will create in your life. This is a bit of a mind fuck when you hear the idea for the first time, and I can hear many of you gasping: 'Lizzy, how the hell do I see myself as something I'm not?'

Well, here's the simple secret: you need to use your imagination and a little of the old 'fake it till you make it'. It may sound scary and impossible right now, but there's a phrase I like, often attributed to Audrey Hepburn, that says 'Nothing is impossible; the word itself says "I'm possible!"' To create change in your life, it's vital that you become aware of the woman you need to become and create a new identity for yourself.

The Exercise

One of my former coaches, Jim Fortin, first introduced me to the idea of living my life backwards (his version is called the 'be-do-have' model[1]) and the following powerful exercise. It's helped thousands of people transform their lives, and I'm confident it will do the same for you.

Essentially, what you need to do is to pinpoint the characteristics and behaviours of the version of yourself who already has what you want.

When Jim told me to do this exercise, I identified the woman with unconditional love for her body is committed to her fitness and nutrition. She works out consistently and regularly cooks and prepares meals for herself that are balanced and healthy. She is courageous when standing up to thoughts of 'not enough'. She acts with integrity by keeping her word to herself as to when she exercises, rests, and takes time out of her day to take care of herself. This is the woman I fearlessly began to embody.

I say 'fearlessly' because fear of failure is a big one for so many women, including myself. However, the woman who harnesses her fear, like the tempest harnessing the storm, will conquer. Let's get brave and ride those waves.

The key to riding the fear is to get quiet. This is also vital to getting clear on your vision. So, get quiet, sit, and take some time for yourself somewhere you can think, somewhere you will not be interrupted and where you can focus and write. You're going to get from this book (and your health and wellness) what you put in, so let's do it from the start.

Ready? Roll up your sleeves. We're living our lives backwards.

Turn to the journal pages at the back of this book—you're going to be using these a lot throughout our work together. On the first page, write down one to three key characteristics of the version of yourself who already has unconditional love for her body. Is she committed, consistent, integral, present, grateful, abundant, aligned, kind, responsible, joyful, loving? Pick traits that emotionally appeal to you. This does not need to be perfect. The list may change or get longer as you work your way through this book.

Next, jot down some of the things this badass is doing. What are some of her daily/weekly/monthly behaviours? You could be doing some of these things already! Whatever they are, they will be specific and impactful in the vision you are creating. They could be physical behaviours like working out three times per week, eating five servings of fruit and vegetables per day, or drinking enough water. Or they could be more spiritual, like trusting, letting go of guilt, and other rebellious acts that I cover in this book.

Finally, how will you feel when you do these things that will get you what you want? Happy, relaxed, calm, peaceful, healthy, strong, sexy, and confident are some of my favourites, but focus on what comes to mind for you. Pick one to three words and note them in your journal.

Once you have this list of characteristics, feelings, and behaviours, you need to read them. Repeatedly. Take five minutes daily when you wake up and go to bed to sit and imagine who this woman is, what she does, and how she feels. Repetition is the master of all learning, and in repeating your goals, you are literally reprogramming your brain with new characteristics, feelings, and behaviours.

The Battle

However, your brain likes your old characteristics, feelings, and behaviours because they are predictable. This predictability keeps us safe—safe but stuck. It is normal that, a few weeks into reading your list, you will start to feel some resistance to doing this exercise and even to some of the behaviours, feelings, and characteristics you originally wrote down.

If you hear your brain telling you, 'Um, no, no, you can't have that', and you feel yourself starting to pull back, *stop*. Tell your brain to calm down and that this is a safe thing for you to be doing.

The solution here is to be more stubborn than your brain, disregard the hesitation, and keep going. It may feel a bit crappy, but this is temporary. What I found, and what you will find, is that after a while—and with constant repetition—your brain will accept the changes you are making and lower the resistance it puts up.

The Summary

Most of us try to achieve unconditional love for our bodies by doing a set of behaviours like working out, drinking plenty of water, and getting enough sleep. This can produce great results, at least in the short-term Yet, over time, so many of us revert to our old ways because we haven't become the version of ourselves who has what we want. We haven't embodied the identity needed to sustain these changes.

This chapter introduced you to the rebellious act of living your life backwards, embodying the character traits and then developing the behaviours of the version of yourself who has what you want. Don't waste time worrying about getting this 'right': what's coming next is going to help you here. For now, let go, have fun, and just start rebelling.

Don't forget to grab your downloadable journal pages at www.nutritionbylizzy.com/journal so that you can complete all the powerful exercises in Reclaim the Rebel with ease and without spoiling your book.

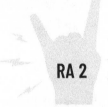

RA 2

REWRITE *your* STORY

Our lives reflect our stories.

Now that you've created a blueprint for living your life backwards, it's time to let go of your old beliefs and create new ones that align with your vision of having unconditional love for your body. It's time to rewrite your story.

The Illusion

Most of us grew up hearing fanciful stories from our family, friends, and teachers that were designed to entertain us. What we didn't realise was that we were being told other made-up stories about every aspect of our daily lives by the same people.

Whether it was stories about money from our parents (a big one in my house was 'you must work hard to get money'), or stories about appearance and body shape from peers in the playground (such as 'being skinny means you are beautiful'), we were surrounded by messages that became embedded in our subconscious belief system. This belief system became solidified over time through experience and repetition, until the stories no longer felt like stories.

Our lives are influenced by a collection of stories we tell ourselves on repeat, formed from past experiences and the stories passed on to us by others. These stories can be positive—for example, I have lived by the story that 'I'm a great dancer' since I was five years old—or negative, such as my long-term story that 'I'm not pretty enough'.

The latter began in the playground when I was seven years old and shaped my life experience up to the age of 30. One day, I was teased that I looked like one of the teachers. The comments made me self-conscious of looking old, having dark circles under my eyes, and of being different from the other kids. I started to tell myself hurtful stories, including comparing my features to someone who'd been in a fight. I hated looking in the mirror and would use every eye cream, gadget, and home remedy I could find to fix my dark circles. I literally tried everything from cold, used tea bags to haemorrhoid cream.

By the age of 11, I was buying expensive anti-ageing eye serums and researching cosmetic procedures to get rid of eye bags. I was so desperate that I was willing to throw money at erasing my perceived flaws to 'finally' become as beautiful as the popular girls.

Around this time, I discovered I needed glasses and used them to hide and disguise my eyes. This shaped my identity as the quiet nerd girl, an identity that remained with me until one December afternoon in 2020 (more on this in the next chapter).

Our lives reflect our stories. If we tell ourselves mostly negative stories about our bodies, what do you think our relationship with our bodies will be like? If, on the other hand, we tell ourselves positive and empowering stories, what do you think the outcome will be?

Psychologist and life coach Dr Linda Humphreys explained this perfectly in an interview with Well+Good: 'the totality of your perceptions ... creates and impacts your personal reality' and these 'perceptions affect the quality of your experience of life'.[2] In other words, if you look at your body through a positive lens, that's what you'll get. On the other hand, if you tell yourself negative stories about your body, you'll be at war with it.

I often see this when working with my clients. When Hannah first came to me, she would tell herself stories like 'my stomach is bigger than my butt', 'I look like an elephant', and 'my boobs look like my grandmother's; they're so saggy'. She also had the story that 'all my friends have had surgery. I should have it too'. She felt like her body needed 'fixing' and was in a constant state of comparison.

Consider your own life for a moment. What are the three most common stories you tell yourself about your body? What is the result of these stories?

Many of your stories will be limiting belief stories about 'not being good enough'. In the previous chapter, we talked about how these stories are total bullshit, and I'm willing to bet they've been robbing you of unconditional love for your body.

Are you willing to have another year—three years, five years—of the same illusion? How do you feel about that?

The Rebellious Act

By now, you should be ready to toss your old stories out of the window as quickly as my grandmother did with her old computer (yep, true story). Similarly, you can probably imagine how radically life-changing the rebellious act of rewriting your stories is. When you choose to tell yourself new, empowering stories about your body, you will see your body in a whole different light.

So, here's a question for you. What are some new stories you can tell yourself that are aligned with your goal of unconditional love for your body? Think of the version of yourself who already has unconditional love for her body. What are the stories she's telling herself? Write these down on a new journal page and save them for our exercise later in the chapter.

It does not matter if you believe these stories yet.

What matters is how far you're willing to go in terms of change. Most people want to change a little, but not completely. This is not rebellious, and it's certainly not effective. In order to reclaim your natural right to unconditional love for your body, I'm telling you that you must be willing to completely transform who you are and what you believe.

Yes, this may feel super scary and extreme (at least, that's how I felt when the idea was first suggested to me), but understand this: if nothing changes, nothing changes. If you don't change who you are and what you believe, you will also not change how much you love your body.

Do not, I repeat, DO NOT, fall into the trap of giving up because of fear and uncertainty. Uncertainty is exactly where you should be in this process. When we're in uncharted territory, we are creating something new. We are creating new stories and new outcomes.

If you try to half-ass this process by sticking to some of the same old stories, you are doing yourself a disservice. This is because you'll be engaging in behaviours and making choices from old stories, which are just going to get you your old outcomes. To get new outcomes, you need to have new stories.

You cannot have unconditional love for your body if you work from the blueprint of your past. Old blueprints produce one thing, whilst new blueprints produce a different result. Keeping parts of the old blueprint will simply dilute your results.

Stop holding on to the handrail, and jump. You've got this.

The Exercise

Beyoncé has one, and you are getting one too. No, not a multimillion-dollar music career that spans three decades. I'm talking about an alter ego.

An alter ego is essentially what we have been creating over the previous two chapters. It's the version of yourself who already loves her body unconditionally. It's all the characteristics, behaviours, and feelings you listed in the last chapter combined with the new stories you're creating in this chapter.

To help your alter ego really come to life, turn to your journal and answer the following additional questions:

- ♥ What is the name of your alter ego?
- ♥ What does she do when she wakes up?
- ♥ What are the things she tells herself?
- ♥ What does she do to look after her body?
- ♥ What does she see when she looks in the mirror?
- ♥ What types of clothes does she wear?
- ♥ How does she feel when she walks into a room?
- ♥ How do people feel in her presence?

Relax and use your imagination.

When I did this exercise, I closed my eyes and dreamt about the version of myself whom I wanted to become. The words just flowed onto the page. Here's what I wrote:

My alter ego is called Grace.

When Grace wakes up, she feels rested, energised, and 100% ready for the day, confident in the knowledge she can deal with anything that she faces with ease. She goes downstairs, makes herself a healthy breakfast, and spends time enjoying a cuddle with her cat whilst looking out the window at the amazing view from her house. She gets dressed in empowering clothes (cute workout clothes or chic office wear with heels), ready for her workout or first client meeting. She looks in the mirror, seeing beautiful eyes looking back at her. She feels pretty in that moment, and she tells herself how fucking sexy she looks and to get what she wants out of today.

She loves learning, especially when it comes to physical matters, and is always looking to improve her skills as an athlete and nutritionist. She takes on new opportunities and challenges and trusts her intuition when deciding what and whom to dedicate her time, money, and energy to.

She never expects anything from anyone but is gracious in receiving compliments. She doesn't worry about being judged, nor does she waste time trying to be perfect. She speaks her mind and isn't afraid of saying 'no' or standing up for herself.

She has regular pampering sessions and works out regularly. She wears minimal makeup and has groomed hair wherever she goes, whether on an important work call or hiking Palos Verdes with her friends.

She loves herself deeply and is so appreciative of her body, mental strength, and energy. She values herself and being with the people she loves. When she walks into a room, people smile. They feel calm and welcome in her presence. She has a nurturing and grounded presence that doesn't ask for attention but naturally draws people to her. She feels completely at ease when in the presence of others and doesn't try to fit in or be impressive—she just is.

So many of the things in my life today, including my confidence, my career, and even my cat, were words before they were ever real in my life. I promise you this exercise works! The key is to give yourself permission to believe that what you envisage for your alter ego is also possible for you and to then train your brain to get on board with this.

After being as detailed and descriptive as possible in your journal, select your favourite phrases from what you just wrote and put them on Post-it notes, save them as notes on your phone, or even make one into a screen saver. Whatever you choose, make sure that your alter ego is highly visible and that you read and think about her frequently. In doing so, your brain will start to accept this new identity and make it your reality.

The Battle

Warning: You may begin to hear yourself say, 'This is silly. I can't do this'. Well—newsflash—that's a story you're telling yourself. And it's a negative story that will not serve you.

What I hope you're seeing here is that our lives are a collection of stories, and what separates those of us with a positive experience in life from those with a negative experience are the stories we choose to tell ourselves.

So many of us have an 'inner mean girl' who loves to tell negative stories, judge and shame us. It is rather shocking, don't you agree, how we women talk to ourselves in a way that we would never dream of talking to our friends and family? Would you ever let your inner mean girl speak to your best friend, mum, or daughter the way you let her talk to you? Hell no! So why let her shame and judge you?

If she starts tapping on your shoulder as you sit down to do this exercise, tell your inner mean girl to go sit in the corner and take her negative stories with her. She can't sit with you at the unconditional love table.

The Summary

In this chapter, I showed you how your whole life is a story that you have created as a result of your experiences of the world. Whilst a kick in the teeth, this is actually really great news. Just as you created the stories, you also have the power to rewrite them and choose different, more empowering stories that are aligned with unconditional love for your body. In fact, the most powerful story you can choose is the one that reminds you that all your thoughts are a story and you can choose any story you want.

Your inner mean girl may be loud right now, so head to www.nutritionbylizzy.com/goodies to get your complimentary Rebel Against Your Inner Mean Girl pdf so that you can quickly learn how to silence her even if you've spent years at war with your body.

RA 3

TAKE *your* GLASSES OFF

I had been forced into taking my glasses off and truly seeing myself for the first time in decades.

Reclaiming unconditional love for our bodies goes beyond changing the stories we tell; it also involves changing how we physically look at ourselves. The lens through which we see our bodies is often so distorted that we need to learn to take off our glasses and view it in a radically new, rebellious way, one that allows us not only to accept but also to finally appreciate how we look.

The Illusion

The sun setting over the water looked particularly beautiful that clear and crisp early December evening. It was no surprise that there were so many people on the Strand in Hermosa Beach. My boyfriend, Steve, and I set out on mile four of our regular weekend run, masked up and COVID appropriate.

As usual, I was going like a bat out of hell and breathing heavily into my mask. My warm breath funnelled upwards, hitting the cold beach breeze and my glasses, forming a fine mist on the lenses. They haven't invented windscreen wipers for glasses yet, so I did the next best thing; I adjusted the side of the frames.

That's when it happened.

SNAP!

The frames disintegrated into my hand.

'Shit' was my first thought. This was a highly inopportune time to not see where I was going. But that wasn't all. I would now need to confront the biggest story I had about my body: 'I'm not pretty enough'.

Remember, this story manifested in many behaviours that robbed me of unconditional love for myself, including using glasses to disguise my facial features and hide. The moment my glasses broke, my perfect plan to conceal my face at all costs also broke.

Anger, frustration, and shame coursed through my veins as we thundered along the Strand. These emotions ran deep and weighed heavily the last three miles of our circuit home. I have terrible eyesight and relied on my glasses all day every day. Even if I'd had 20/20 vision, I couldn't have seen anything as

I cried my eyes out when we ran up the driveway and reality began to hit.

I had been forced into taking off my glasses and truly seeing myself for the first time in decades.

The Rebellious Act

Although I was cursing the universe for a week as I adjusted to living life with contact lenses, it was during this week that I discovered probably the most powerful rebellious act in this book, the act I had been seeking since I was an eleven-year-old kid searching for solutions to my under-eye dark circles. This did not come from a cosmetics store or plastic surgeon. It came from my coach, Sara Drury, teaching me how to stand up to my inner mean girl and her stories in the mirror.

I stood staring at my reflection for an uncomfortable amount of time. I looked for the good in what I saw. You know, kind of like Luke looking for the good in Darth Vader in *Star Wars: Episode VI*. But there was nothing. All I could see were the dark circles under my eyes. I tried reciting several positive stories other people had told me in the past: I have nice blue eyes and beautiful, long eyelashes. The stories felt unbelievably hollow.

I returned to the mirror the next day, hoping the result would be different. I had the same empty feeling as I told myself the same stories, but this time I had to fight back tears of frustration. 'Why don't I love myself?' I whimpered.

Determined not to be bullied by my inner mean girl, I did the same mirror exercise again the following few days. Again and again, I couldn't seem to say anything nice about myself.

On the sixth day, I was about to give up on the whole process when, suddenly, I heard myself mutter, 'I have good skin'. Shit! It was finally working.

The next day I came back. 'I have beautiful thick hair'. Oh, that felt kind of good.

You know what I did? That's right! I kept it going.

For two weeks, I did this mirror exercise and took a daily selfie. Over time, I created more and more nice stories about my body and believed in the compliments I received. I was also able to reframe the negative stories and stop my inner mean girl in her tracks before she started whispering illusions of 'not enough' in my ear.

I made myself even more accountable by posting the photos I took in a private group of my friends on social media.

My first post read:

The reason for my anxiety. My face. I avoid mirrors, photos, and get triggered by people who are 'beautiful'. My glasses broke last night, so now I have to wear my contacts, something I've avoided for years. I make up stories about not being sexy or pretty and just hide myself. I've considered cosmetic surgery to 'fix' my face. I don't want to feel this way. So, I'm letting go of that starting today and promising to post a photo of my face every day [for the next 14 days]. Here's day 1.

On the 14th and final day, I posted again with a montage of the two weeks' photos with the caption:

Two weeks of self-love selfies! Thank you so much again for all the love and support. Is it any coincidence that last night I dreamt I helped unlock secret places where people were living but had no idea existed?! I'm so ready for [next year].

The Exercise

The mirror exercise was conceived by the mother of self-love herself, Louse Hay, and has since been adopted by thousands of women all over the world. Although it's not easy, this exercise was beyond powerful for me, and I guarantee you will find it just as powerful.

Remember Hannah from the last chapter? In combining the mirror exercise with the alter ego exercise, she was able to change her stories about her 'saggy boobs' and 'squishy stomach' to empowering thoughts about her body's curves. She no longer wanted surgery like the rest of her friends and started to embrace her natural beauty. When she looked in the mirror, she saw her alter ego and began posting confident, sexy pictures of her body online.

Whether you've been hating on your thighs or your nose, I encourage you to look in the mirror or even take a photo of your body daily. Look at yourself for a period of time that is uncomfortable for you, such as five minutes, and just observe.

What stories are coming up for you?

Is there anything nice you can say about your body?

How can you reframe the negative stories to be more empowering and aligned with having unconditional love for your body?

For example, you may really dislike your stretchmarks after giving birth, but what if you looked at your stretchmarks as a sign of how incredible your body is to have grown a little human inside of it? What if you looked at your stretchmarks in awe?

I have a big scar across my stomach that made me super self-conscious whenever I wore a bikini. This scar was from life-saving surgery I had as a baby when my small intestine telescoped in on itself. When I began to practice having more self-love, I reframed my story about my scar and saw it as a sign that I was strong. It became my survival scar.

The Battle

My inner mean girl was very judgemental when I first did this exercise. You will probably find this as well. She may tell you how vain it is to be looking in the mirror or to care about your appearance. She may try to divert your attention to the parts of your body she knows you find hardest to love.

These are all tactics to keep you stuck in the same thought loops and habits. As I explained in chapter 1, this doesn't seem to make sense until we realise it's a mechanism to make life predictable and therefore 'safe'. But we don't want safe. We want to rebel against the bullshit and get out of our perceived comfort zone because that's where positive changes happen.

Even if you feel like this is fake or clichéd, it takes you a while to get used to, or you start to feel discouraged if you don't immediately feel more confident, keep going anyway. That was the best advice my coach gave me about this exercise. She shared how it took her a while to get used to it when she first started and how she didn't believe any of the words she was saying to herself either. In fact, she 'couldn't even get the words out' to begin with. 'I would just stand there', she said.

Believing nice things about our bodies can be hard for a lot of women. However, as model, body activist, and fellow mirror exerciser Ashley Graham emphasises: 'It doesn't come overnight, but if you keep working at it, eventually you'll believe it.'[3]

What really helped me was having a cheer squad of friends for this exercise. Cheer squads are awesome, and I'll explain why later. I didn't want to let these people down, so even on days when my inner mean girl started to get the better of me, I took the damn photo and posted it in the group.

And that's the most important point behind this whole chapter: take the photo, look in the mirror. Make like a Nike ad and just do it. When we are 100% committed, our lives are much easier because there's no thinking involved. Being 99% committed, by contrast, is so much work. We have this internal battle over whether we do or we don't. When we 'umm' and we 'ahhh', it wastes so much of our finite energy. Why not make it easier on yourself by going that extra 1% and fully committing to the rebellious acts that will help you reclaim unconditional love for your body?

The Summary

In this chapter, I introduced you to probably the most powerful tool for changing your stories about your body: the mirror exercise. It requires full commitment to confronting your inner mean girl. When you do this, you will begin to change your self-image within a matter of weeks.

Words can't fully describe what a total game changer the mirror exercise is in helping us appreciate our bodies, regardless of how long we've been struggling with accepting our appearance. Therefore, I simply encourage you to try it for yourself. Repeat after me: 'mirror, mirror, on the wall …'

In chapter 12, you're about to discover how awesome having a cheer squad really is. In the meantime, head to www. nutritionbylizzy.com/squad to join my wonderful community full of free tips and support for your journey to feeling good in your body.

RA 4

PUT *yourself* FIRST

In order to help others, we need to help ourselves first.

A massive paradox is that we as women are so good at loving others but fail miserably at loving ourselves. Dove's Self-Esteem Project found over half of women admit to being 'their own worst beauty critic'.[4] Shockingly, the National Institute on Media and the Family reports that by the time girls reach the age of 17, 78% are unhappy with their bodies.[5] Moreover, seven in 10 girls surveyed by Dove say they won't be assertive in their opinion or stick to their decision if they aren't happy with the way they look.[6]

Low self-worth is a widespread issue that needs to be solved *now*. So, I'm going to make an audacious proposal: we need to recognise our value and put ourselves first. What does that even look like when we have a full-time job, two kids, a stressed hubby, and ageing parents? Well, my friend, let me tell you.

The Illusion

Anyone who has ever boarded a commercial aircraft has heard this basic instruction:

'In the event of an emergency: put on your oxygen mask first before helping others'.

It makes sense that, in order to help others, we need to help ourselves first. This applies to emergencies, but it is also essential in our daily lives.

However, most women are brought up with the story that they should put themselves last. A dear friend and client, Jessica, summarised the feeling of guilt we can experience if we put ourselves first: 'It feels so unnatural and a bit selfish'.

Being seen as selfish is the last thing most of us want. On the other hand, it's almost like a badge of honour to be the self-sacrificing martyr. The problem is, this causes low self-worth.

I've seen this in my own life. My beautiful mum, for example, is often praised for being the most caring, kind, and selfless person, but I also saw as a kid that she didn't value herself.

It was subtle, but I noticed. For instance, whenever we would buy food at the grocery store my mum would always get the cheapest option available for herself whilst Dad and I had whatever we wanted. When she served up chips for dinner, she would always give herself the blackened burnt ones, or she'd eat the broken biscuits from the packet and leave the 'good ones' for everyone else. We absolutely loved going clothes shopping together (and still do), but whilst she would insist she had to buy me the items I liked, she would never buy herself anything. Even that gorgeous £7.99 nail polish was an extravagance for her.

Putting other people and things before my own needs was also how I lived my life for many years. For example, instead of sleeping, eating well, and relaxing with friends, I would work myself to the bone when I was a student.

Are you also someone who always puts other people and other things before your needs?

This could be a symptom of low self-worth and could be damaging your mental and physical health. You may become resentful of others and feel disconnected from your relationships.[7] This was me. I had no time for people I cared about and didn't make the friendships I craved as an undergraduate.

Physically, it may cause malnourishment, issues with eating,[8] and ultimately result in burnout. For years, I had a pattern of burning out from work, which meant that I had to rest and other people had to look after me. However, as soon as I had recuperated, I would do the same thing again.

The last time I did this, I was the only student in my nutrition MSc class who graduated in the summer. This was because I had to delay sitting for my finals due to burnout from over studying and perfecting. I didn't make time for sleep. I was so hell-bent on getting top marks that I would study until exhaustion, so much so that I compromised even getting a degree.

Standing alone on stage at graduation, I realised I needed to learn the act of valuing myself.

The Rebellious Act

I had my 'aha moment' in regard to how to value myself after reading Gary Chapman's *The 5 Love Languages*.[9] It's a great read, and I highly recommend that you check it out.

The premise of the book is that there are five different ways we communicate love (the five love languages): physical touch, words of affirmation, acts of service, quality time, and gift giving. Once we identify our primary love language and our partner's primary love language, we can use this to nurture and deepen our romantic relationship. The idea is by using their love language, we effectively communicate our love to our partner.

The 5 Love Languages got me curious. What if I could turn the concept around and use my primary love language on myself to communicate unconditional love for my body?

Turns out, my primary love language is receiving gifts—not really a shocker considering I love Christmas so much! I therefore started experimenting with my theory by going on a solo shopping trip.

Until then, I rarely spent money on nonessentials, so it was beyond exciting to gift myself workout clothes and cute jewellery. I felt so valued despite the simplicity of the exercise.

The Exercise

Of course, what floats your boat may be completely different. Therefore, I would encourage you to play around with this.

Start by asking yourself what your self love language is. Do you like it when people pay you compliments (words of affirmation)? Or do you feel loved when someone gives you a hug (physical touch)?

Here are some suggestions as to how to use your self love language. Your assignment is to do at least three of these this week and share which ones you choose by tagging @ NutritionByLizzy on your Instagram page with the hashtag #MySelfLoveLanguage. I encourage you to get creative and find ways that make you feel valued.

Words of affirmation—write yourself a love letter (which you can read back as you progress on your self-love journey), have a 'self-appreciation' box on your desk that you add to daily, write nice things about yourself on Post-it notes and hide them around the house for you to find at a later date, or programme words of affirmation into your phone calendar as reminders that go off throughout the day.

Physical touch—go for a massage, cuddle up in cosy blankets, wear soft/comfortable clothes, give yourself a facial, or have a luxurious bubble bath.

Receiving gifts—buy yourself flowers, take yourself on a shopping trip and buy yourself a gift (it doesn't have to be expensive, but if it is, that's even better), buy yourself lunch out as opposed to making it at home, gift yourself a vacation, or upgrade yourself to first class when you travel.

Quality time—take the day off, spend some time alone reading/doing crafts/painting/playing a musical instrument, call your best friend to have a chat, or take yourself on a date.

Acts of service—organise your wardrobe or desk, make yourself a nice dinner, or hire an Uber or taxi to drive you to your next appointment.

The Battle

This probably all sounds very exciting. I mean, who wouldn't want to feel valued? The best part is that you get to be the one who does it, in a way that resonates with your heart! All you need to do is figure out your self love language. Take the 5 minute quiz at http://www.nutritionbylizzy.com/quiz.

The main challenge with this rebellious act comes when we have competing values: the kids, the husband, the elderly parents, the job—these also matter to us. When we add in other things and people that we value, it can become difficult to balance everything simultaneously.

When Jessica reached out to me, she knew she was struggling with balancing her home life with her wellbeing and needed help. She wanted to care for her kids and husband and keep the house looking spotless, all whilst juggling a full-time job. She also wanted to be healthy, yet she was having trouble with this because she was prioritising everything and everyone else in her life over herself. She didn't make time to sit down to eat a meal and instead was fuelling her body with just the kids' leftovers, coffee, and an occasional cereal bar here and there.

We prioritise what we value. Therefore, it's important to commit to making yourself a priority, even with these other factors in play. This is where you need to take one step further in flexing your self-worth muscle. Reorganising your schedule by putting activities that intrinsically show your value first and doing everything else second is a powerful way to do this.

Personally, this equates to making myself a healthy breakfast and having 'me time' at the beginning of the day without checking emails. During this time, I might do a workout. Another day, I might go for a walk to buy myself a latte from Starbucks—using my primary love language.

This is all about creating something that works for you and your life. Therefore, I recommend you create a list of things that you can pick from at the beginning of each day, things that you enjoy doing and that will help you feel valued. A few ideas include:

♥ journaling or writing out things you're grateful for (more on this later),

♥ reading a chapter of a book with an empowering message,

♥ listening to a podcast you enjoy, or

♥ taking a long shower.

When I was first introduced to the concept of putting mysef first every day, I was horrified. If you baulk in horror at the idea of doing this, like I did, you are right where you need to be. Remember: discomfort is the zone in which change happens.

Let me reassure you—the world won't stop spinning, the kids won't tear down the house, and your boss won't fire you for prioritising yourself. What I found instead was that I felt more energised, still got my work done, and was in fact a better partner as a result of reorganising my day.

My clients have seen outstanding results also. Jessica went from always putting others first to taking time out of her day to make herself nutritious meals and practice yoga. As a result, she now feels so much calmer, her skin and digestion have improved, and she has gained a whole new level of confidence— so much so that Jessica is now considering changing careers, something that she says would never have happened had she not learnt to prioritise herself.

I hear you asking, 'But Lizzy, what if I forget to reorganise my day? I'm in the habit of doing my day this way, not that way?' That's an excellent question. I'm asking you to change a massive habit by putting yourself first in your daily routine.

I've found using a habit tracker super useful for this. A habit tracker is simply a tool to keep track of the daily habits you want to form, from having a healthy breakfast to stretching for ten minutes to taking a walk around the local park.

I like to write things by hand, so my habit tracker is a piece of paper with daily habits listed in chronological order that I tick off as I go. I put my tracker in a prominent place where I cannot avoid it (i.e. on the wall above my desk). Other good places to put a habit tracker include on your mirror or on your fridge. Head to www.nutritionbylizzy.com/goodies to download my favourite habit tracker.

If you are technologically inclined, there are also tonnes of great online habit trackers and apps that work along the same lines, sending you automatic reminders and allowing you to tick off your habits as you complete them. Find something that works for you.

The Summary

In this chapter, I encouraged you to make the rebellious act of putting yourself first. Reorganise your day and practice your love language on yourself as ways of increasing your self-worth. Far from selfish, this will not only benefit you by nurturing unconditional love for your body but also everyone else around you.

You know self love is important, but reading about it doesn't mean there's change. That's why I'm about to actually guide you through the process using my simple two-step Self Love Language Method™. Head to www.nutritionbylizzy.com/quiz to discover how to boost your self love even when you're busy.

RA 5

Be VULNERABLE

Vulnerability is the courageous act of connecting with others about our life story in order to show our authentic selves.

The last couple of rebellious acts are powerful, life-altering tools that will benefit your inner peace and energy levels. However, they also require a great deal of vulnerability.

It's important to be clear on what vulnerability is. Some of us have numbed out our vulnerability for so long that we can't even recognise it or are afraid of even 'going there'. But this is a book about being rebellious, so I'm going there.

The Illusion

I love how Brené Brown discusses the topics of authenticity, courage, and connection as well as what gets in the way of these crucial elements of vulnerability. I highly recommend adding her book *The Gifts of Imperfection* to your reading list.[10]

To paraphrase, she explains that courage, connection, and authenticity are essential for living a joyful life with unconditional love for ourselves. However, shame and judgement are barriers to practicing vulnerability.

Shame essentially keeps us quiet, and judgement keeps the inner mean girl playing on repeat in our heads. The illusion is that being vulnerable is a weakness, when in fact vulnerability requires courage.

I hated being vulnerable. For example, shame would prevent me from sharing the fact that I suffered from an eating disorder years after I had recovered. I remember being shamed at school when it was first made public that I had anorexia nervosa. One of the girls in my class announced to the room how she felt 'disgusted' by my condition. This felt like a knife to the heart and put me in shame for the next 14 years.

I also feared being judged. I would torture myself with: 'What if they judge me for being a nutritionist? What if they are judging me for what I'm eating? What if they start judging me for my shape and weight?' This kept me closed off and precluded me from building deep connections with others in my personal and professional life.

The Rebellious Act

The rebellious act here is to recognise shame and judgement, push them aside, and be vulnerable anyway. The key is not to ignore but to acknowledge and then dismiss the feelings that get in the way.

For me, it was like learning to become like my best friend, Louise, who stood by me throughout my eating disorder. Whenever other girls at school would make a mean comment, she would defend my corner. She could have easily shrunk into the background and ignored these situations, but instead she acknowledged what was happening and put her vulnerability on the line to help me. Therefore, when I started practicing this rebellious act, I would think about Louise and draw on her strength.

It also helped me to remind myself that judgement is inevitable. Humans will always judge. This judgement can be positive, such as 'this is a really great book' or negative, such as 'she took way too long to publish it'.

People are going to judge no matter what. And who cares? What matters is what you know in your heart to be true. I know some people may disagree with my outlook, but I am living my purpose and speaking my truth, and that is all that matters.

It's actually selfish of me to give into my fear of judgement. I'd be keeping my story to myself and not sharing what has finally allowed me to love my body unconditionally. Consider how many people I can assist by sharing my story, opening up, and being a vulnerable, flawed human. Imagine how many people *you* can help by being vulnerable about your experiences.

The important realisation I had when reading Brené Brown's work was that shame loves perfectionists. It keeps us in line by playing on our desire to look perfect on the outside—cool, calm, shiny, bright, and squeaky clean—basically, wanting our life to look like a perfectly polished Instagram feed. On the inside, we are peddling a million miles an hour to keep up this perception, and when we can't (which is inevitable), we feel shame.

To overcome perfectionism and shame, we need to accept ourselves as human, with real emotions and imperfect lives. In other words, we need to practice being vulnerable by showing our emotions and telling our stories.

This is *big*. Being vulnerable for a lot of women can mean opening the floodgates to waves of emotions they haven't allowed themselves to feel in a very long time and remembering parts of their lives they have swept under the rug. Mentally, it can be tough to take the leap and ride the wave for the first time. But as with anything new, it gets easier with practice.

When you begin to practice being vulnerable, start small with people you trust the most. This is because it will help you feel safe to let it all out, including the tears. Crying is a physical outlet of emotion, and sometimes that outlet, just like the outlet on a pressure cooker, needs to be released.

The problem comes when we stuff our emotions back down as soon as they start bubbling up. By stuffing those emotions down like a bulimic going on a cookie binge, we are hurting our bodies. In the short-term, it can literally lead to binges or using food for emotional support. In the long-term, it can lead to chronic disease, weight gain, and depression. The solution is to let yourself feel all the things—good, bad, and ugly.

This is something that I held back from for a long time. I felt like I had to always be perfect, which included never showing vulnerability, dark emotions, or fears. But I had a lot of these—especially as an anorexic teenager—that needed to be shared.

Two years into my illness, I was at a breaking point. My self-destructive patterns were beyond the scope of my community care team, and I had only gained a few pounds since I was first diagnosed at 14 years old. I felt frustrated, misunderstood, and constantly under surveillance.

This night was no different. As I sat at the living room table, silently pushing dinner around on my plate, I could feel the steely eyes of my parents watching me. Then came my opportunity: Dad nipped up to the bathroom, and Mum popped out to the kitchen. I grabbed my dry, anaemic-looking food and shoved it into the nearest thing I could find: my graphic design portfolio. My parents entered the room again and were impressed—although a little surprised—that I'd finished my meal.

'Ha, gotcha', I thought.

A couple of hours later, we were watching TV. When the cat trotted passed my portfolio, his nose twitched. Within an instant, the twitch went into overdrive.

I froze as Dad jumped up to investigate. As he peered in my portfolio, I prepared for the disappointed look on his face.

'Oh, Bun'.

'I'm so sorry', I pleaded.

I waited for Dad's next phase of grief: anger. He was often angry those days. 'Baby, I get why you did that. You wanted prove you could eat'.

A part of me melted. That was the first time I felt understood by anyone during my illness. It was also the first time I felt I was on the same team as my parents: Team Bun. This team became incredibly powerful from that day.

Indeed, my family was fundamental throughout my journey of developing unconditional love for my body.

I realised this as I sat alone at my computer one January afternoon, tears welling in my eyes, as I proofread my nan's eulogy. My memory flooded with the times I used to drive her nuts when I was five years old and insisted on fiddling with my hair. She always said I looked beautiful.

I didn't realise until 25 years later, sitting 5,000 miles away from where she once lived, that she had taught me the most valuable lesson: that my imperfections are actually perfect. At that moment, I realised my beauty and power were not in how I looked. They were in my vulnerability and willingness to be me. I hope that one day you, too, will see this in yourself.

Take it from me—quit the need to be perfect. It's total crap. Give yourself grace. Feel like crying? Let yourself cry. Feel scared about being vulnerable? Share with those you trust.

The Exercise

There are in fact many ways to practice being vulnerable. The biggest thing that helped me was sharing more of myself on social media. This involved the selfie exercise I mentioned in chapter 3, as well as doing more vulnerable posts and videos where I shared my story of the eating disorder I had suffered as a teenager. After realising that my clients and prospective clients didn't know the whole truth about why I am a nutritionist and why I love what I do, I decided to finally open up about it.

I first posted about my history of anorexia on my business page. It read:

Why am I a nutritionist?

… and why my answer surprises me.

In the past, I would have said something super vague like 'because I want to help people stay healthy and live life to the fullest'. And that's true.

However, this is masking my true 'why', which I've always been hesitant to share for fear of putting myself out there and being judged. That is until now.

Truth is, I struggled with a 10-year eating disorder starting at the age of 14. My grandad suffered from a range of health issues and then died suddenly from a heart attack (16 years ago yesterday in fact). I didn't want that to happen to me, so I turned to magazines to 'learn' how to be healthy. My naivety combined with their bad advice resulted in the exact opposite, and I became dangerously ill.

It took so long for me to fully recover, but when I did, I found my purpose.

I am deeply passionate about what I do, and part of sharing that passion is being open about my own journey. I want to speak more about this—as well as eating disorders in general—but first I'd love to get your feedback: Is this of interest? What do you want to hear about? What don't you want to hear about? I'm now open to being open, and helping you out is always worth fighting my own fears and insecurities. So go ahead, comment below, or if you'd prefer, private message me here, via email or text.

I felt mild discomfort as I hit the 'share' button on my post, but it also felt good once I had done it. At that point, sharing on my business page was the baby step I needed to take.

Once I had made this step, it became easier to open up. For example, I started doing live videos on social media and sharing more experiences. It snowballed quickly, and now I'm writing this very vulnerable chapter in this very vulnerable book.

My challenge to you is to first identify a vulnerable experience or story that you want to share. It could be something about your past that you've never told anyone or even something that happened recently that made you feel vulnerable. Then, find a way to share your experience that feels mildly uncomfortable, whether that means talking with your partner or best friend or sharing a post on social media. Finally, be courageous and share this experience or story without the fear of being judged.

It's important to remember that it's about taking baby steps here. Mild discomfort is what we're aiming for, not pain. Too much vulnerability too soon can be overwhelming, causing you to retreat into your comfort zone rather than moving forward.

The Battle

We've lost our sense of what it means to authentically show who we are, what we're feeling, and to share our experiences as a society. Allowing ourselves to be open and honest requires a great deal of courage and to let go of that perfectionism I mentioned earlier.

It still scares me to open up and share at times, but what's great about fear is that it's all in our heads, which means we have the power to deal with it. When I feel fear, that's when I examine my stories around being vulnerable and practice being courageous instead.

The truth is that sometimes we have to take the initiative and share first. However, I've discovered that the most personal things are often the most general. As a result, for every one person who shares, there are a slew of others who have had similar experiences. They may not take the risk of sharing this publicly, but they do benefit from the courage of that one person who does.

The advantages of opening up far outweighed my expectations. I never expected that—in being vulnerable myself—I would have so many other people share their own stories and experiences. Some of my adult friends shared how they, too, had suffered from an eating disorder when they were younger, which I would never have known if I had not shared my experience. Other women sent me DMs sharing how much the idea of an 'inner mean girl' resonated with them. From there, we discussed techniques on how to silence her.

In essence, sharing my story and being vulnerable normalised our collective experiences. It created the sense that 'I am not alone in this' and built a whole new level of connection that I couldn't have envisaged.

The Summary

I'll be real with you here—I found this chapter super difficult to write. That's because topics like vulnerability, shame, and judgement are things that most of us generally try to avoid. If we hide from them and allow our fear to get the better of us, we close ourselves off from making deep and meaningful connections by showing our authentic selves. It takes plain courage to put our vulnerability on the line, but when we do, the results are pretty extraordinary.

By now, you're probably starting to think 'wow; I can totally relate to what she's been saying'. If so, I'd love to connect with you further. Head to https://bookme.name/lizzycangro to book a complimentary connection call with me. No expectations or agendas; just 20 minutes to connect over coffee (or your favourite beverage).

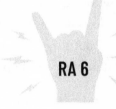

RA 6

FORGIVE *yourself*

Self-compassion is a highly rebellious thing to practice. It involves allowing ourselves to move gently towards what scares us or causes us emotional pain.

Oh my goodness, I've just realised something. We're halfway through our journey together! I've shared some hugely powerful rebellious acts and you're beginning to witness for yourself how life changing these can be. This may feel like a gutsy move—and you must trust me on this one—but you're now ready to forgive yourself.

The Illusion

It may not seem obvious that you need to forgive yourself,

but let me ask you this question. Have you ever told yourself off for something you have done and then continued to beat yourself over the head with it?

Yep. Me too, girl.

In fact, one of my most vulnerable, perfectly imperfect experiences on my journey to achieving unconditional love for my body is one that I had not forgiven myself for until very recently. I haven't shared it publicly until now.

I was only 16 years old and a few months out of the hospital from being treated for my eating disorder. It was a Thursday evening, and I was doing the weekly family food shopping with my mum.

'Can I get Evian water again, please?' I asked Mum as we went down the drinks aisle at Tesco. 'The bigger bottles?' I was a fancy anorexic. I was also desperate.

The deal I'd made with the hospital was that I would be weighed every week. This was to prove that I had been eating enough and therefore was maintaining my weight. Ideally, though, I would have been gaining weight.

But the truth was, I had not been eating at sixth form college. I threw out my sandwich every day before I left for my train journey, leaving a few crumbs in my lunchbox for creative effect.

In order for me to conceal my drop in compliance (and consequently my weight), I drank water before weighing in. But not just a little water. I'm not even talking a glass or two. I would down three to four 750 ml bottles of Evian beforehand.

How did I manage this? I picked my weigh-in day to be a Tuesday, the day I had a free period in the afternoon, so I could go home early and drink all my water before Mum got home. I would try pacing myself as best I could by starting on the train and finishing in my room, before jumping on Mum as soon as she got in the door to ask her to weigh me. By this point, I was desperate for the bathroom and couldn't hold it in much longer.

Drinking too much water, a.k.a. water intoxication, can decrease blood sodium to extremely low levels. In some cases, this can lead to seizures, coma, or even death.[11] I was completely oblivious to the dangerous behaviour I had developed until one Tuesday when I felt so sick and so dizzy after I had been weighed that I had to run out into the garden to hide from my mum's inquiring eyes. I was terrified she would find out my secret.

For years, I felt like I'd not only failed at staying well, but I'd also failed my parents. The key to freeing myself from the regret and guilt I felt was to forgive myself. To do this, I had to learn self-compassion.

The Rebellious Act

Self-compassion is a highly rebellious thing to practice. It involves allowing ourselves to move gently towards what scares us or causes us emotional pain. This is the exact opposite of our natural response to self-protect. There is also a tonne of vulnerability involved, and we now know how tricky that one can be.

I found being kind to myself extremely difficult. In fact, I coined the term *pull-up mentality* to describe my lack of self-compassion.

The phrase *pull-up mentality* came about one afternoon during a workout with Steve. It was back and triceps day, and as usual, we were doing pull-ups as part of our routine. I was grunting and moaning as I began to fail on my last rep. 'One … more … nope'. I started to descend into all the negative self-talk and bullshit I used to tell myself about not being enough.

Steve just smiled, shook his head, and handed me his phone. He had taken a picture of my back without me realising whilst I was doing my set. 'You are strong: just look at those back muscles', he said. 'Stop bullying my girlfriend'.

From then on, we started using the term *pull-up mentality* to describe my mindset whenever I started beating myself up, whether it be about my workouts, my face, or my body. This phrase was a reminder that I am enough and to practice being gentle with myself.

A few months later, I was blessed to come across inner-child work and started using it in place of pull-up mentality to achieve unconditional love for my body. This is the healing practice of pausing to tune into that younger version of ourselves that we lose touch with over the years.

To rediscover my inner child, I found a picture of me wearing a princess costume my mum had made. I was five years old, still little and cheeky, with blonde hair and big innocent eyes.

I also thought about the games Little Lizzy would play and what she liked to do. I remembered where she went on holiday and what her favourite outfits were. The more I thought about her, the more I connected with Little Lizzy. I could feel myself smile as I heard Little Lizzy get excited about going for a walk to the beach and getting ice cream with me.

It may sound a little quirky, but that's the point. Connecting with our inner child is so.much.fun!

It's also so powerful for practicing self-compassion.

Instead of judging myself, I would begin to ask, 'Would I talk to my inner child the way I'm talking to myself right now?' The answer was always a resounding 'no'. That's when I would ask, 'What does Little Lizzy really need to hear?' My answer would then dictate what I said to myself or did next.

I would tell myself (and still do) that I was doing the best I could and that no one is right all the time. I mean, just think about it: whilst at school, 100% on a test meant you were acing the class; 100% at life probably means you are a robot. (Cue: Little Lizzy doing a robot dance!)

The Exercise

It's time to free both yourself and your inner child from the grudges you've held against yourself, some of which you may have been harbouring for a really long time.

Turn to your journal and ask yourself, 'What can I forgive myself for?'

Start making a list. It can be as long or short, detailed or general as you like. It may include small stuff, like forgetting to defrost the meat for dinner and having to get takeout, or big stuff, like using exercise to punish your body (see chapter 8 for more on this). Make a list that resonates with you and don't overthink here.

My forgiveness list went something like this.

I forgive myself for:

♥ The years I wasted obsessing over calories

♥ Putting my body in danger by being so underweight

♥ Putting my body in danger by drinking so much water to hide my low weight

♥ Defining my worth by my appearance

♥ Worrying about a number on the scale

♥ Lying about eating

♥ Throwing food away

♥ Using exercise to burn off calories

♥ Not asking for help when I needed it

♥ Being hard on myself when I was struggling

♥ Wasting my money on magazines to tell me what to eat

♥ Depriving my body of the nourishment it needed

♥ All the stuff I put my parents though when I was anorexic, including the stress and time they spent trying to get me well

Next, I want you to really feel the emotions that come up as you write. Maybe you feel fear, regret, guilt, shame, frustration, or even anger. What resonates with you? Close your eyes and really go deep. It's okay—you've got this.

Finally, and with your eyes still closed, I want you to imagine your inner child. Use an actual photo of yourself as a child if it helps. Visualise holding this little girl's hand, giving her a hug, and saying, 'I'm sorry. Please forgive me. Thank you. I love you'.

Now open your eyes.

The Battle

This is one of the tougher exercises in this book, and it's likely you will feel some resistance, especially to feeling the emotions you need to feel in order to forgive yourself. For example, you may be experiencing regret and guilt similar to what I described earlier; these feelings, along with most other emotions you will feel when writing your forgiveness list, are uncomfortable.

However, it's important to sit with the discomfort so we can process and move through the emotions we haven't fully dealt with. For example, regret and guilt are unhelpful feelings we get from continuing to live in the past. Living in the past prevents us from living in the present, and although you can't change your past, you can release it and the accompanying emotions that reside there.

Of course, this is where self-compassion and the inner-child piece of the exercise are vital. What also helped me was burning my list. You may want to practice the above exercise several times before doing so (and when you do, do it as safely as possible), but take it from me: burning my list felt so freaking good and totally rebellious. Try it for yourself. Even better, take a video, post it on your social media page, and tag @NutritionByLizzy with the hashtag #RebelOnFire.

The Summary

The fact that you are doing the work and having breakthroughs whilst reading this book means there is a need to forgive yourself for all the years of physical and mental self-abuse. This chapter showed you how to do this through developing more self-compassion and connecting with your inner child.

Forgiveness is an important, yet overlooked, element of self-love. It is the rebellious act that sets you free from your past so you can live in the present and finally find peace within yourself.

Remember those cute party bags we used to get as kids? Well, fun and feeling good are my top values so I've decided to create my own FREE goodie bag just for you. Head to www.nutritionbylizzy.com/goodies

RA 7

TRUST *your* GUT

Self-trust means we are trusting ourselves with our choices.

It won't come as a surprise that, as a nutritionist, my clients come to me with all their nutrition questions. This is fantastic because I absolutely love answering questions. However, half of the time my clients already know the answer. So why ask? The real reason they ask and invest in my services is because they don't trust themselves. This is something that, in addition to developing their nutrition knowledge, we work on. It's vital you do the same, so this chapter is going to be dedicated to learning the rebellious act of trusting your gut.

The Illusion

That day was just like any normal mild, slightly dreary summer Tuesday in northern England. I was staying with my dad's parents on the opposite side of the country and, like any other 14-year-old grandchild, enjoying the delights of my gran's cooking and being spoilt by my grandpa.

However, that all changed in the early evening when my dad walked through the door. He had a solemn look on his face. Deep down that's when I knew something was wrong. Indeed, that evening my whole life changed.

'Sit down, Bun', Dad said.

'What's going on?' I interrupted.

'I wanted to tell you in person. This morning, Grandad passed away from a heart attack', he whispered.

I felt like my own heart stopped at that moment.

My mum's dad, my grandad, had battled Parkinson's disease, lung cancer, and now this?

In all the head rush, I couldn't help wondering if I had anything to do with him dying. You see, about three days beforehand, I made my grandad his favourite dessert, lemon drizzle cake, to help him feel better through his latest round of chemo. I feared I could've somehow poisoned my grandad with this cake.

That is the first memory I have of not trusting myself with food.

I began to look for advice on nutrition in magazines and on websites. The more I looked, the more I didn't trust myself with food. I thought I needed other people to tell me what to eat. This meant I adopted some terrible advice (including to exclude dairy products from my diet), leading to an unhealthy relationship with food and, later, my 10-year battle with an eating disorder.

Ironically, as an anorexia patient who wanted total control over what she ate, all my food decisions were taken away from me. Once again, I was relying on other people to tell me what to eat to be healthy. This felt totally suffocating and disempowering. It was also freaking confusing. My care team's advice was completely different from what I had read in the magazines. Yet, both made me feel like I was eating for purpose, not pleasure. I never enjoyed food; nothing from the crisp crunchiness of an apple to the silky creaminess of dark chocolate made me excited.

It was only when I was working a midweek shift at my job at Starbucks and felt a painful pull in my lower back that this started to change.

I feared what this pain in my lower back might be, so I went to my doctor. She referred me to the hospital to get a bone scan. The results were devastating. It revealed that, at the age of 22, I had developed osteoporosis (severe bone loss) in my lower back. This is hardly surprising since from the age of 14 onward, I had excluded dairy products from my diet, and dairy is a vital source of bone-strengthening calcium. My osteoporosis was something I was told I could never cure and that I needed to be careful when lifting, as I was at an increased risk of fracturing my spine.

I certainly didn't identify as someone who had a condition normally associated with post-menopause. I therefore began to learn about nutrition from official sources of advice like the National Health Service (NHS) and British Nutrition Foundation, determined to finally kick my anorexia to the kerb.

In fact, I was fully recovered from my eating disorder within a few years of taking responsibility for my health and decided to pursue a master's in nutrition at King's College London. This helped me expand my knowledge and, as a result, trust in myself.

I started going to the gym to learn how to lift weights and stopped taking the calcium supplements that my doctor had prescribed to help slow any further bone loss. Instead, I prepared balanced, varied meals that provided my body with all the nutrients it required.

As of my last bone scan, I had gone from having osteoporosis (the most severe type of bone loss) to osteopenia (a less severe version). My eyes welled up when I opened my scan results; I had finally learnt to nourish my body and trust myself with food.

The Rebellious Act

Let me ask you this: how much of your time, money, and, quite frankly, wellbeing have you wasted on bad advice, fad diets, and diet pills over the years?

I wouldn't be surprised if you have invested hundreds, if not thousands, of dollars in your lifetime. According to Yoni Freedhoff in his book, *The Diet Fix*, the weight loss industry has grown to be a $66 billion industry, yet at least 90% of diets fail.[12]

The heartbreaking thing is, so many of us have given our power to individuals and companies that don't want us to love ourselves. If we loved ourselves, we wouldn't need them anymore, and they wouldn't make money from us. If you trusted yourself to make healthy, balanced choices, you wouldn't need to buy into their bullshit.

How much more of your hard-earned cash are you willing to give away to fund the diet industry?

Learning to trust yourself by taking responsibility for your health and wellness is the key to breaking free from its shackles. When we take responsibility, we are acknowledging that we have a choice.

Self-trust means we are trusting ourselves with our choices.

I've been there. I know it's scary to trust yourself with the decisions you make over food. You were, however, born with the intrinsic ability to nourish yourself. Your body's functions are so elegant and sophisticated, including letting us know when we're hungry, full, or require more of a certain nutrient. Ever craved chocolate when you're on your period? Well, that's your body signalling to you that it needs a feel-good pick-me-up of carbohydrates.

Another excellent example is the wonder of our liver in naturally detoxifying substances within our body. As a result, you don't need to do a cleanse. Trust me, they are a waste of time and money. They can also lead to nutrient deficiencies and, in the case of juice cleanses, cause unhealthy spikes in your blood sugar. Yes, the marketing is attractive, and the packaging may look nice on the refrigerator shelf, but that's the nicest thing I can say about cleanses.

Be rebellious and turn your back on this crap. Toss all your little bottles and, instead, learn to trust yourself, whether that's eating carbs or having a small glass of wine with dinner. Not only will you feel better within your body, you'll be nourishing your bank balance.

The Exercise

Warning: learning to trust yourself with food requires time and practice. This is certainly not an overnight, one-and-done thing. The secret sauce is deciding to be 100% committed to the process and being kind to yourself throughout.

Making the decision to listen to and honour what your body is telling you is one of the most important things you can do. This can be accomplished in several ways, but start by tuning into something as basic as your hunger levels. When you're unsure whether to eat and how much, rate your hunger on a scale of 1–10.

1. I'm ravenous—I could eat my own limb.

2. I'm hangry and have no energy—don't mess with me.

3. I can't hear you—my stomach is growling.

4. I'm a little peckish, I guess.

5. I'm 50/50—neither hungry nor full.

6. I'm mostly satisfied.

7. Ahhhh. I feel pleasantly full.

8. I'm gonna sit down for a bit—I'm full and slightly uncomfortable.

9. I feel stuffed like a Thanksgiving turkey.

10. Uh oh—I feel sick.

If you are a four or below, eat something. Stop when you reach a seven.

I also love setting daily alarm reminders on my phone that encourage me to trust myself. It's a simple tool, but a consistent reminder helps me stay on track with my eating habits. I can choose to binge out of a jar of peanut butter with a spoon, to keep working and skip lunch, or to have a limp salad that is in no way appealing for my dinner. But are these really what I want to choose? It's up to me to be responsible for making the best choice for my body. The more I listen to my body and honour what it tells me, the more I trust myself with these choices.

What's vital when you are reclaiming responsibility for your food is to stop blaming your circumstances and other people. Whilst certain situations and people can be more conducive to helping you love your body, ultimately the buck stops with you.

Sure, having an unsupportive partner or limited grocery budget is not ideal. However, you've still gotta eat, girl. You can nourish yourself on a budget, for example, by buying in bulk and stocking up on canned food. You can also stop mindlessly grazing on snacks with your partner.

What do you choose? Do you choose to live by circumstance and put you and your health last? Or do you make the choice to reclaim your right to unconditional love for your body?

The Battle

Ultimately, with learning to trust yourself with food, you need to go within and ask yourself what your body needs. However, I also understand the genuine need for clarification and support with some areas of nutrition. This is where working with a qualified nutritionist and knowing where to look for reliable information is invaluable.

For example, a lot of people ask me about the keto diet (as well as other diet fads out there). This is something that I generally do not recommend, and when I explain to clients why carbohydrates should be around 45%–65% of our total energy,[13] I tend to get suspicious looks. Carbohydrates are our body's preferred source of energy, and not having enough in our diets can lead to brain fog and lack-lustre workouts.

I love hearing how, after eating more whole grains, fruits, and veggies, my clients have so much more energy. For Carolina, the difference was noticeable within days. She loves cooking traditional Spanish dishes but was concerned that they were too carb heavy. When I explained that carbohydrates would in fact help her tennis performance, she began to include more within her meals, especially on days she trained. It was so rewarding to see her beaming with energy the next week as she reported how much better she had played.

These 'aha!' moments are great, but they also highlight a challenge with learning to trust yourself with food. The sheer volume of information out there can set you on the wrong path with your nutrition, suck you back into questioning your choices, and confuse the hell out of you.

The key is to know how to wade through this information. You can use your gut instinct in this respect, but you can also look at who is giving this advice and decide from there if you trust them.

The title *nutritionist* is not protected by law (unlike *dietician*). Therefore, please be mindful of this, especially on the internet and social media. When deciding whether to work with a nutritionist or even when reading an article, my tip is to be on the lookout for certain letters after that person's name.

There is a voluntary register, called the Association for Nutrition, of qualified professionals with degrees in nutrition from British universities. These people can use the letters ANutr or RNutr (Associate or Registered Nutritionist) after their name. I'm on this register. The letters RDN (Registered Dietician Nutritionist), meanwhile, signify those who have gained degrees in nutrition and dietetics from an American university.

Working with a qualified professional can enrich your knowledge and further your self-confidence. My aim is that clients never need me after six months; by then they trust themselves enough to nourish themselves with their food. To me, that sounds so much more freeing than being stuck in the hamster wheel of the diet industry for the rest of your life.

The Summary

This chapter feels closest to my heart out of all the rebellious acts in this book. When I finally took responsibility for the choices I was making, I gradually learnt how to trust myself with food and achieved unconditional love for my body. This rebellious act gave me back my time, money, and health. It also led to a more balanced and sustainable approach to nutrition where I can now relax, enjoy food, and get on with my life. This rebellious act is the only diet you'll ever need to invest in if you want the same for your body.

If you're someone who's exhausted by cycling through all the diets out there and looking for a plan that actually works for YOU, head to www.nutritionbylizzy.com/intensive to book a 75-minute Rebel Intensive. In this 1:1 call with me, you'll come away with a personalised step-by-step action plan that works for you and your lifestyle so that you can easily and effectively make the changes you need to feel good.

MOVE FOR *pleasure,* NOT PUNISHMENT

Just like how we choose our thoughts, how we choose to move our bodies matters.

Before we get started, I have a confession to make. This chapter was written to the sound of ABBA's 'Dancing Queen'. The fact of the matter is, I absolutely love dancing, and this song always reminds me of that. Dancing is something that brings me so much joy and taps into my creativity and playfulness. It's a perfect example of what moving for pleasure looks like. So, on that note (no pun intended), let's dive into this rebellious act.

The Illusion

When I opened my business, I got a lot of my clients through referrals from personal trainers and gyms. The reason is that people most commonly associate having their dream body with exercise. My clients would go to their trainers first if they wanted to change the way they looked and felt. The trainer would then bring me in to assist with the nutrition aspect, which is just as important as exercise (if not more so).

Exercise, like food, is something that has the potential to be used as a tool for self-abuse. This was evident in the clients who were referred to me, as well as in my own personal experience.

As a kid, I loved to dance (ballet, tap, even Irish dancing—you name it, I tried it). To me it wasn't exercise—it was fun. When I was about seven years old, I moved to a school with acres of fields. I realised that my love of playing in the dirt combined with my long legs made me a decent cross-country runner. This was the first time I was aware that I was 'exercising'. It didn't bother me, and I found a lot of joy in running. What did bother me was when we had to play netball. Even worse, cricket!

Fast-forward to secondary school, and suddenly, I was the only girl who still liked to run (or at least was the only one who would admit it). I was good at it and enjoyed the competitive element of representing my school. I had given up dancing because in my mind it wasn't 'cool' to be a dancer. Running was so much more mature.

'Oh, and look, it's also super healthy. This magazine said so. And it burns calories? That's good, right? Ah, and I'm good at it, which means I'm proving the boys wrong when they're making fun of me for being a nerd'. These were all the thoughts that were the makings of my unhealthy relationship with exercise.

Looking back, it was the perfect storm for me to use running as a form of punishment. It looked something like this: I would have a bad day at school where someone was mean to me. I ran to 'run away' from my feelings of inadequacy. It gave me a hit of endorphins, and I felt better. It was kind of a 'fuck you, I'm good at this' feeling. I'd then get compliments at school because I was getting better and better at it, so I kept running more and more. As I continued to do it, I started to get skinnier and skinnier because I didn't know how to use food to fuel myself. Again, I would get 'praised', this time because I was getting thin. Finally, girls liked me because I had the body they wanted, and boys gave me respect because I was good at sports. All this external validation kept me literally running myself into a very unhealthy place.

The day it all stopped was when I was diagnosed as anorexic.

I don't quite remember how they managed it, but somehow, I found myself in a doctor's office with my parents. I probably don't remember because at that point, I felt as if I'd been tricked out of an afternoon of classes and after-school cross-country.

In protest, I had decided I would save my lunch until after the appointment. As the nurse went in to take my blood, a part of me regretted my decision. See, I've had a phobia of blood all my life and pass out very easily at even the mention of it. I'd been passing out at school in my biology classes recently, and I didn't fancy doing the same now. To my relief, this nurse didn't take my blood. She couldn't even find a vein.

So, the doctor tried himself. And he tried again. And again. It would have been easier for them to get blood from a stone; it would have had more life to it for sure. How do I know this? Well, my heartbeat was around 30 beats per minute, and my blood pressure so low it was in the Antarctic. I was dying. I was anorexic.

Wait, I was what???

The only other time I'd heard of this condition was in the girls' changing rooms after PE. There were giggles as one of the girls accused another of being anorexic because she didn't want a piece of candy.

'That's not me', I thought.

The doctor's words echoed in my ear during the whole drive to the hospital. The only time I couldn't hear his voice was as I stuffed my sandwich down my throat.

Once we got to the accident and emergency department, everything was a blur until I was told that I was banned from doing any form of movement. I wasn't even allowed to walk. I was warned that if I kept doing what I was doing, I was at risk of dying from a heart attack—the very thing that triggered my eating disorder. My awareness went into overdrive in that moment, and I handed over my running shoes right then and there.

Although I was physically prevented from doing any exercise whatsoever and couldn't act out my unhealthy behaviours, inside I was no different. The connection between exercise and self-abuse had been solidified and lay dormant throughout my eating disorder.

What prevented me from working out when I had anorexia (and for a long time after I had recovered) was the extreme fear of having a heart attack. I was terrified at the thought of overdoing it and keeling over at any moment. Memories of the day my grandad died flashed through my brain any time I contemplated moving my body. Even running for the train gave me panic attacks. For me, this time in my life represented the other extreme of the spectrum that many women experience with exercise—not doing anything, not trusting our bodies, and living in fear.

After learning about my osteoporosis at the age of 22, my stubbornness to finally rid myself of my disordered thoughts and behaviours was even greater than the fear I had of exercising. With my doctor's permission, I started to do exercises that would help me with my condition.

I dipped my toe in the water by going to a Pilates class. Whilst I was totally scared, both of moving and of being the newbie, I felt a glimmer of achievement at the end of the class and soon became a regular attendee.

However, remember that dormant volcano I mentioned earlier? It was still there. It was only a matter of time before I started pushing myself a little bit more … and a little bit more.

Back at university, I felt confident of my body's ability to cope with movement. I was also struggling a lot with my postgraduate course (I was training as a teacher, which I absolutely hated). The pressure of university meant I searched for an outlet to make me feel better. This was partying, drinking, and working out. I remember being so tired from pushing my body that I could barely stay awake on the first day of my school placement. I was back to my old pattern of self-abuse. This time, it was the adult version.

The Rebellious Act

I despised feeling so exhausted, the guilt of missing a workout, and the constant feeling of going through the motions. Instead, I wanted to enjoy working out, just like that little girl who used to dance along to 'Dancing Queen'. I decided to make a new choice.

Just like how we choose our thoughts, how we choose to move our bodies matters.

I was fortunate to be introduced to the Cambridge Dancers' Club whilst I was a student. This group held Latin and ballroom lessons at local venues around the city. One of my good friends at university discovered how much I loved to dance and asked if I'd like to go check out a class. I avoided going for a couple of months, but he persisted in asking. I'm so glad he did.

When I finally gave in and went, I had the time of my life. It was like stepping right back into being 10 years old, smiling and giggling and having a tonne of fun moving my body to the beat of the music.

It was this dance class that showed me how to enjoy exercise again. I had so much fun dancing with my partner, learning cool new moves from my teacher, and walking out of each class feeling like I was on cloud nine. It was only then that I noticed I was glowing, not only from happiness but also from sweat!

The Exercise

Moving your body for pleasure—not punishment—is all

about how you feel and trusting yourself to decide what is right for your body. Therefore, take five to 10 minutes today to stop and really think about the types of movement that bring you pleasure (and yes, all types of movement count here). From a gentle yoga session to a full-on dance party in your living room, make a list in your journal so you can pick from it whenever the mood to move takes your fancy.

Here is my list:

- ♥ Dancing! Whether it's at a party, in my living room, or taking a dance-inspired workout class
- ♥ Doing a gentle yoga session
- ♥ Going on a run by the beach with my partner
- ♥ Going on a walk surrounded by nature whilst listening to music, a podcast, or audio book
- ♥ Working in the yard

To me, music and movement go hand in hand. So, as an extra tip, I suggest making a playlist to work out to. Again, I've provided a few of my favourites below:

- ♥ Spice Girls – 'Spice Up Your Life'
- ♥ S Club 7 – 'Bring It All Back'
- ♥ Britney Spears – 'Stronger'
- ♥ Five – 'Keep On Movin' '
- ♥ Destiny's Child – 'Bootylicious'
- ♥ Peter Andre – 'Mysterious Girl'
- ♥ Hanson – 'MMMBop'

♥ Backstreet Boys – 'Larger Than Life'

♥ NSYNC – 'Pop'

♥ ABBA – 'Dancing Queen'

Give me cheesy pop, and I'm in my happy place. I have no shame in admitting this. But I want to know about you. What's on your list? Head to social media and tag @NutritionByLizzy with your top tunes.

The Battle

Dance is a tough thing for a lot of people to enjoy. This is because it is full-on, total-body vulnerability. The only other version of this is being naked, and we all know how vulnerable that can feel. However, I believe deep in my soul that dance is part of being human. Children dance with pleasure on their own accord until society tells them a story about it not being cool and that they should be concerned about how they look and what other people think.

Comparison and fear of judgement are huge barriers to allowing yourself to move for pleasure rather than punishment. Dealing with this is a whole other rebellious act that's coming in chapter 11. For now, let me explain how this may manifest itself in the specific context of exercise and how to move past comparison in an instant.

You might be boogying your heart out at a party or shaking your booty at your weekly Zumba class when you notice your attention shift from your fancy footwork to your head. You start telling yourself stories like 'I look silly', or 'She is much better at this than me'. Yes, that's right—it's your inner mean girl again.

Send her packing with four simple steps:

Step 1: Notice that you are doing this to yourself.

Step 2: Stop it. Literally just stop.

Step 3: Keep dancing and shift your attention back to the music and your happy feet.

Step 4: Repeat if necessary.

I must admit, after joining the Cambridge Dancers' Club, it would be another seven years and a lot of practice in the four-step process above until I was able to break the old patterns I had developed as a kid.

This is also an area where I worked on building self-compassion. I told myself that it took me three years to develop an unhealthy relationship with exercise and 10 years of sustaining it, so seven years of breaking out was to be expected.

I had periods of being extremely critical of myself for not having it all figured out, but I also had periods of listening to my body and trusting myself. Over time, the healthy behaviours outnumbered the unhealthy until one day I looked around on one of our runs and realised I was no longer trying to prove or punish myself. I was moving because it felt good. And that felt really good.

I've since run a half-marathon with Steve and a couple of our other friends at a pace that felt comfortable for my body. Passing the 13.1-mile finish line was an exhilarating feeling and a major milestone in my journey. I was ecstatic for the girl who was told not to move a muscle because she could die, who got so wrapped up in trying to prove herself, and who used exercise for all the wrong reasons.

The Summary

Many women have lost the feeling of joy and excitement when it comes to moving our bodies. It tends to evaporate when we are teenagers for a variety of reasons; the most common is that we become more conscious about our changing bodies and what other people think. This can result in our losing interest in movement altogether. In my case, I was the opposite—I went overboard with movement.

Although they are on opposite ends of the spectrum, neither situation fosters unconditional love for our bodies. But what does? Dancing in your living room to your favourite song, letting go, and being goofy. Try it tonight, and I guarantee it will make you smile and bring a spark of joy. You go, Dancing Queen!

Ready to move for pleasure not punishment? Get your dancing shows on and head to www.nutritionbylizzy.com/goodies for my favourite feel good playlist. No sign up or subscription is required.

RA 9

EASE *up*

Rest is essential for our biological functioning; it allows for mental and physical recovery and replenishes our energy levels so we can be our best selves.

Can I let you in on a little secret? When I first read the title of this rebellious act, my nose twitched a little. Why, you may ask? Because rest does not come naturally to me. Ironically, I've had to work incredibly hard to stay focused on this area of self-care and in the process learnt a lot about rest, which I'll share with you here. Listen up to ease up.

The Illusion

What do I actually mean by rest? For the purpose of this

chapter, rest is defined as sleeping, sitting still, and slowing down to do things for the sake of doing them.

Sleep is the most common type of rest that I discuss with clients. This is because getting enough quality shut-eye is vital for regenerating our minds and bodies. Yet, as a society, we are hugely sleep-deprived.

Research suggests this has both short- and long-term consequences for our health. People who don't get enough sleep are at an increased risk of heart disease or stroke, compared to those who sleep seven to eight hours per night.[14] Meanwhile, individuals sleeping less than six hours per night have repeatedly been shown to be at an elevated risk of type 2 diabetes.[15, 16]

Sleep deprivation also disrupts daily fluctuations in appetite hormones, including increasing levels of ghrelin—the hormone that stimulates hunger—and reducing levels of leptin—the hormone that suppresses hunger. This is believed to cause cravings and poor appetite regulation.[17]

Unfortunately, many of us pooh-pooh the idea of sleep and believe it is a luxury. We don't consider its benefits and instead perceive it as a sign of laziness. I came to believe that sleep was an extravagant use of my time and would force myself to stay up beyond the point of tiredness when we were hanging out with our friends. I didn't want to look like the delicate princess who needed her beauty sleep. So, I would push through, despite not having any energy, and force myself into having a good time, usually with the assistance of alcohol.

The next morning, I would feel groggy and be super quiet. I hadn't given myself the time I needed to recharge, and my body always paid the price. My relationships also suffered because I didn't have the energy to be my usual fun, bubbly self. Instead, I was short and moody with the people I loved the most.

I remember one time, coming back from a soccer tournament in Las Vegas with Steve, our flight was at 6:30 a.m., and we had gone to bed at 2:30 a.m. that night. As our plane taxied onto the runway, I burst into tears. I was beyond the point of tiredness and felt so resentful for having stayed up so late when I knew we had an early morning flight. I was not taking care of my needs or taking responsibility for my choices.

After Steve held me for the entire flight and during the Uber ride home, I collapsed on the bed while he got ready for work. Alone, and with a thumping headache, I knew something had to change. That something was me.

In addition to depriving myself of sleep from fear of judgement, I also used exhaustion as a sign that I was working hard enough. This was especially an issue for me as an undergraduate at university, where I would compare myself against how hard other students in my class worked.

If one of the girls was in the library before me, I would get in an extra hour earlier the next day. If I heard one of the boys had pulled another all-nighter, I would have to do one too. My inner mean girl would tell me to suck it up and push through it whenever I felt tired. By the time I finished my finals, I was exhausted, stressed, and existing—not living.

I craved achievement, thinking that once I had accomplished it, I could slow down and catch up on sleep. But, with this mindset, I never could ease up because I never felt like I achieved enough. As a productivity addict, things like sleep, sitting still, and 'doing things for the sake of doing them' were so foreign and stressful to me, I felt like I was wasting my time. If it was not on the to-do list, it wasn't important to me.

Can you relate? Are you able to slow down, or are you also always on the go?

The Rebellious Act

Rest is essential to our biological functioning. It allows for mental and physical recovery and replenishes our energy levels so we can be our best selves. This is a win-win in terms of work, relationships, fitness, and overall wellbeing.

The biggest thing for me was believing these benefits. I was sceptical, but when I made sleep a priority, I saw that my world didn't fall apart. It actually got better. This meant I could allow myself to let go of the need to be 'on' every waking hour of the day.

I also let go of the fear of judgement. I learnt to stop caring about what other people thought about how hard I worked and what time I went to bed. I became very adept at declaring, 'I'm done for the day. It's been real. See you in the morning'. And being okay with that.

Learning how to rest provided me with another opportunity to practice self-compassion. I had to silence my inner mean girl who wanted me to just keep going. This is where knowing how to manage my anxiety and being still was key.

Initially, I thought stillness meant meditation, and to be honest, meditation just sounded so freaking awful. Sitting crossed legged and quiet for hours, trying to think about nothing, sounded like torture. However, I realised that stillness could mean different things to different people, from meditation to breath work to praying.

I found that what worked for me was taking 30 minutes daily to practice self-hypnosis, an exercise that slows our brainwaves to a more relaxed state.[18] I have an audio recording that I listen to every morning before I get out of bed and every night before I go to sleep, and it's totally revolutionised how I view stillness. Stillness used to be a pain in the butt, but now I view it as an absolute essential.

Whatever method works for you, a regular practice of quietening your mind is so necessary for easing up and feeling a sense of inner peace. It creates a space for you to breathe and be calm, all whilst sleeping a hell of a lot easier. This means you have more energy and don't need as much caffeine to get through the day.

Rest is more than just being still and having adequate sleep: it's also making time for the activities you enjoy but that don't necessarily lead to anything productive. It could be as simple as playing with your kids, watching a movie, or doing something creative. It could also be taking the time to prepare a meal or going on a weekend getaway.

This type of rest provides expansion in our lives as well as an opportunity to play, which is something we as adults tend to lose sight of. However, playing is the fast track to creating more joy in life. It can lift our spirits and help us reconnect with our inner child as well as create better relationships with those around us. For example, I get very giggly and goofy when I start playing. Not only does this make me feel lighter, it also makes me a fun person to be around.

The Exercise

This rebellious act requires you to take time out of your busy day. So, put your feet up and turn to your journal. Spend five to 10 minutes making a list of things that you like to do 'just because'. Anything that brings you joy.

For me, my 'just because' list looks something like this:

- ♥ Going on a walk by the beach in Hermosa
- ♥ Sitting on our roof-deck in the sunshine
- ♥ Cuddling up with our cat on the sofa
- ♥ Watching a chick flick (*Legally Blonde* is my all-time favourite)
- ♥ Hanging out with our friends at home and playing pool in our garage
- ♥ Going on a weekend trip to Big Bear
- ♥ Calling my best friend and parents in England
- ♥ Cooking and baking for my American family (visit www.nutritionbylizzy.com/recipes for a few of our favourite recipes)
- ♥ Playing a board game (we love Harry Potter and Ticket to Ride)
- ♥ Doing a jigsaw puzzle
- ♥ Doing some sort of craft project (for example, at Christmas I make cards and Christmas crackers)

Got your list? Good. The next bit is the fun part. I want you to now rebel against your to-do list today and instead pick something from your 'just because' list. Have fun and lose yourself in your 'playtime' for however long you want, be it 15 minutes or a couple of hours.

Want to really ramp up your 'easing up' game? Start to experiment with ways to be still. Start by just sitting still for half an hour. No music, no phone or electronics. Just sit with yourself and notice how it feels.

Finally, make a conscious decision to go to bed 15 minutes early tonight and set your alarm to go off 15 minutes later in the morning. Think you can do this for the whole week? Of course you can! Use your habit tracker to keep you committed so you can get 30 minutes of extra sleep per night. In seven days, that's an extra three and a half hours of rest!

The Battle

Sitting still and resting present something of a paradox. They are essential antidotes to anxiety, but they also are highly anxiety provoking.

The reason why so many of us struggle with easing up is the fact that in doing so we must face the reality of our lives (i.e. that we are exhausted and need to rest), and that feels uncomfortable. Very uncomfortable.

You're going to be making some changes to your day, and in doing so, you're going to feel resistance not only from yourself but also from those around you. Everyone will have been accustomed to you running around like a headless chicken, so when you make changes to slow down, some people may ask if you're doing okay. This comes from a place of genuine concern and love for you.

However, whatever you do, don't crumble and go back to your default setting just to prove that everything is fine. Stand your ground and explain how you're making changes in your life—that includes easing up a bit and enjoying more downtime. You are responsible for your choices, not their reactions.

You may be able to do the above, but deep down, it may also feel terrifying. You may start asking, 'What if I'm wrong? What if slowing down means that the spinning plates fall? What if busy and exhausted is what it takes?'

Well, my friend, what if you're not wrong? What if rest is exactly what you need? What if you're well rested and happy? If this matters to you, then choosing to make this rebellious act is vital.

Take a breath and trust yourself here.

The Summary

We need to take more time to slow down, to play, and to sleep. When we first start to do this, it can suck, especially if you're of an anxious disposition. However, with practice, your ability to relax becomes easier, and you will start to notice the benefits to your overall energy levels, relationships, and sense of wellbeing. You'll begin to rebel against the grind and reclaim yet another part of unconditional love for your body.

One of my favourite things to do to let go of the hustle and ease up is listening to a podcast. In fact, I've found podcasts so useful in my own wellness journey that I've been spreading the rebellious word on topics in this book. Head to www.nutritionbylizzy.com/podcasts to check out my eclectic mix of conversations and discover new shows to listen to.

DRESS *up* (OR DOWN)

In order to have unconditional love for our bodies, we need to be okay with showing up and being seen for the beautiful women we are.

My love for dressing up began when I was six years old. My mum worked for a bridal company that did fashion shows. I was the designated bridesmaid every weekend, which essentially involved getting my hair styled, wearing pretty dresses, and being paid in wedding cake. It was the best.

In fact, rediscovering how much I enjoyed dressing up was a key piece of reclaiming unconditional love for my body. Let me explain why it's also going to be important on your journey.

The Illusion

Have you ever worried about your clothes, hair, nails, skin, or makeup? I'm talking anything from whether your clothes look good on you to seeing your first grey hair to deciding what shade of lipstick to wear.

Have you ever worried about worrying about your appearance? This includes judging yourself for stopping at the mirror to check how you look or being afraid other people will think you're vain.

If you answered 'yes' to either of the above, you're not alone in having anxiety about your appearance. Like many of the other illusions I discuss in this book, these fears begin in childhood when we are taught that the way we look matters but also that it's important not to care too much about the way we look. It's a lose-lose situation.

My earliest memory of this was when I was nine years old and getting ready to go to a birthday party. At that age, I loved wearing dresses, doing my hair, and wearing as much sparkle as possible (this was the '90s, so I totally embraced the body glitter)!

However, that evening I was agonising over whether to wear my favourite midnight-blue party dress because I didn't have a bag that matched.

Standing in front of the hallway mirror, I was anxious that my friends wouldn't like me because I didn't have clothes with matching accessories or that I didn't look as put together as they did.

My grandparents, who were taking me to the party, were

starting to get impatient with my indecisiveness.

'You've got to be careful; you'll end up being vain', my nan whispered as I got in the car.

By the time I turned 10, I owned just one dress and didn't care about dressing up anymore. I wasn't having nearly as much fun, but at least I wasn't vain. Throughout my teens and 20s, I continued to buy into the illusion that caring about what I looked like meant I was vain.

This all changed when I realised that there is nothing inherently wrong with vanity (so stick it, inner mean girl) and that it was the intention behind my beauty routine and how I dressed that really mattered. For years, I was choosing my clothes and beauty routine out of fear, when in fact the key is to come from a place of self-love.

I know a lot of women who won't let themselves dress up or down for fear of being judged. Some women feel the need to wear a whole beauty counter on their face. They get up earlier than the rest of the house to put it on so their partner and/or kids don't see them in their natural state. Others worry that wearing makeup will make them appear overdone. Some women cannot bear to be seen in a hoodie and sweats, whilst others fear that they won't be able to walk in heels.

So much fear.

By now, I don't need to tell you how suffocating fear is. In the context of how we adorn our bodies, fear can prevent us from expressing our true selves. The intention is to keep us safe, but as we know, safety is not always conducive to self-love.

The Rebellious Act

In order to have unconditional love for our bodies, we need to be okay with showing up and being seen for the beautiful women we are.

The goal is to have a routine and wardrobe that are aligned to our goal of showing unconditional love for ourselves. For some women this means dressing up every day; for others it means forgoing makeup completely. It's entirely up to you how this looks.

Personally, I love looking after my skin by cleansing with a basic micellar water and applying moisturiser with a rose quartz facial roller (neatly, rose quartz is associated with self-love). This takes about five minutes of my day, and it makes me feel really good. I tend not to wear makeup—I just curl my eye lashes and give them a swipe of mascara. That's enough for me.

I enjoy spending a little more time and money on hair care, so I geek out on luxury brands like Living Proof and Christophe Robin (which Steve refers to as my 'Winnie the Sham-Pooh'!). I take my time in the shower to shampoo and condition my hair as well as use the occasional hair mask. I'll treat it with heat-protecting spray, blow dry, and finish off using straightening irons to tame any flyaway strands.

I paint my nails every week and tend to choose the same shade of red for both my toes and fingernails. I love matching colours! I also love wearing red—it feels so empowering!

Clothing-wise, I'm a comfort-loving creature and tend to live in yoga pants, sports bras, and trainers. These tend to be solid colours, with very little detail or patterns. I wear a lot of black, as well as blue, both of which I like because they bring out my eyes and compliment my skin tone.

If I'm going to a party, I'll go all out with a dress and heels. Again, these will not be overly detailed or patterned but instead will be solid colours that have interesting lines or shapes woven into the design.

The way I dress and use beauty products fully represent me as a person. I can say hand-on-heart that I don't care in the slightest if someone else doesn't like the way I look because I know I'm being true to myself. That's really the goal of this rebellious act, to forgo how you think you should adorn your body and instead embrace clothes and a beauty routine that reflect you and make you feel good.

The Exercise

Turn to a fresh page in your journal! Write down what comes to mind when you think about the intention behind your current routine and wardrobe. Are you coming from a place of self-love, or are you still operating from a place of fear and judgement? Where do you need to make changes so your clothes, beauty products, and makeup are aligned to your goal of reclaiming unconditional love for your body? Really take some time here to reflect.

When you have fully assessed where your current intention is and where changes need to be made, the next step is to close your journal and open your wardrobe, bathroom cupboard, and makeup bag. Let's to do a radical audit!

Go through each, one by one, asking yourself whether what you currently have is in alignment with you feeling good about your body. If your answer is a confident 'yes'—it's in alignment with feeling good about your body—then keep it. If it's a re-sounding 'no', it needs to go! Put it in a pile to give to a girl-friend, sister, or niece next time you see them. Anything they don't want you can donate to charity.

Look at all that extra space you've made!

Now that you've made room, it's time to have some fun! Re-visit that journal once more and make a list of what clothes and beauty products are in alignment with having unconditional love for your body.

What can really help as you craft your vision is to think back to the alter ego exercise we did together in chapter 2.

What would your alter ego wear? How does she do her hair? Does she paint her nails? Think in terms of colours, textures, shapes, fragrances—it all counts.

Next, and this is the best part (especially if your primary love language is gift giving), take yourself on a shopping spree and buy items that are on your list!

The genius in this is that not only are you filling your life with items that are more representative of you as a person but you are also rewarding yourself for all the amazing work you've done during our time together. This provides recognition and signals to your brain that the changes you are making are safe.

The Battle

You may not have very clear answers to the above questions. That's okay. Relax, breathe, and allow your thoughts and ideas to flow naturally. The key is to have fun and not overthink this. Equally, it's not a race, so if you do want to let your brain mull it over for a bit and come back to this exercise after a few days, that's fine too.

You may also feel completely overwhelmed at the thought of doing this exercise for your whole wardrobe and beauty routine. Whilst I highly advise that you go big with this rebellious act, I never want you to feel like this is too much too soon. Remember, do what feels best for you.

Instead, why not just start with one aspect of your wardrobe or beauty routine? Maybe you go through your makeup bag and throw out the free foundation samples that don't match your skin tone. Maybe you discard the nail polishes that are thick and goopy or have begun to separate. Or maybe you go into your underwear drawer and throw out all the off-white panties, socks with holes in them, and underwire bras that dig into your ribs.

When you go shopping, you can also start small. Make an appointment at your local beauty store for a foundation co-lour-match session, or buy a matching bra and panties set in a colour you love to wear.

The latter is my secret tip to feeling good every day. Since the age of 16, I've worn matching underwear, and whilst no one else but my partner gets to see, it makes me feel put together, confident, and sexy. This means, in turn, that I give off a totally different vibe, leading not only to a better relationship with my body but also with my partner.

Whatever you do, be careful of falling into the old trap of devaluing yourself. Give yourself permission to buy new clothes, makeup, and beauty products. If you are worried about the financial implications of buying yourself these gifts, start small as above—it's okay to take baby steps. If you still feel uncomfortable, you may want to review chapter 4 about prioritising yourself.

The Summary

Dress up, dress down—it's your choice. The intention is to use your beauty routine and clothing to show your body gratitude and love. You are beautiful either way, so choose to adorn your body in a way that makes you feel good and is aligned with your true self. Who cares what anyone else thinks?

In this chapter, I mentioned several of my favourite products and practices for dressing up (or down)! Find more product recommendations and receive exclusive discounts by heading to www.nutritionbylizzy.com/discounts

LET GO *of* COMPARISON

Trying to 'measure ourselves up' against other women is putting a gauntlet of scales, tape measures, and mirrors between us and our happiness.

Throughout this book, I've addressed some massive barriers such as fear, judgement, and shame. I'm now going to expand on this by discussing how comparing ourselves to others is a major form of judgement that robs us of our joy and inner peace. It's undeniably a barrier to achieving unconditional love for our bodies, and that's why I'm going to teach you the rebellious act of how to let it all go. Spoiler alert: it's super simple but highly effective!

The Illusion

Humans are social creatures, and as social creatures, it is very natural for us to observe what other people are doing, what they look like, and how they dress. Knowing about and conforming to social norms has helped humans throughout history form and maintain groups, and these groups helped our ancestors survive.

However, comparing ourselves to others has its downsides. It's very easy to get sucked into a negative spiral of judgement. This is something I call *shoulding on ourselves*. Common examples include 'I should look like that', 'I should dress like this', and 'I should be that weight/shape/height'.

Something that I used to should on myself about—a lot—was my pale skin. When I first started dating Steve and moved to SoCal, I was beyond self-conscious that I didn't have the sun-kissed glow that most Californians seem to have. I told myself the story that in order to fit in and be attractive, I should have a tan. You know, less 'Casper the Friendly Ghost' and more 'Baywatch bombshell'. Therefore, I would get weekly $49 spray tans to cover up my skin and feel more confident around the locals, including Steve and our friends.

When the COVID-19 pandemic hit, my illusion shattered. I couldn't get my tan because the salon was forced to close. Yes, I could DIY it, but I tried that once and ended up looking like a rare Californian zebra! Hardly the blending in I was going for! I was so stressed about the whole thing that I even developed a rash.

So, there I was, standing naked in the shower in front of my boyfriend of 18 months, pale and pasty and with a massive red rash. There was a lot of shoulding in that shower. I felt so exposed and just wanted to hide under long sleeves and track-suit bottoms.

Shoulding on yourself (whatever form it takes) is literally like piling a tonne of crap onto yourself and burying your unique-ness under comparison. This is not practicing unconditional love for your body and instead is a recipe for perfectionism, anxiety, and low self-esteem.

Trying to 'measure ourselves up' against other women is put-ting a gauntlet of scales, tape measures, and mirrors between us and our happiness.

If you try to quantify how skinny, pretty, tall, toned, and tanned you are, using others as your benchmark, you will al-ways feel like shit. This is because, in a world of billions of women, it is inevitable someone will have what you don't. And then what?

I spent decades of my life comparing my body to other wom-en's. Not only did comparison keep me feeling like I wasn't good enough, and kept me spending money on products to fix myself, but it also had dangerous implications for my health.

When I was released from hospital all those years ago, it was on one condition: that I eat. As I mentioned in chapter 6, I would be weighed in each week, and if I was not holding up my end of the bargain, I would be put back in hospital. I was de-termined not to go back there. I would do anything to prevent that from happening.

Motivated as hell to prove my care team wrong (my dad had

to convince them I was ready for this), I trotted off to sixth form college with meals, snacks, and backup snacks. 'I'm going to do this', I insisted.

I was so excited about my new start, and this excitement attracted a lot of new friends. Finally, I was popular and healthy and free! The free part was, however, to be my downfall. I hate to say it, and please don't tell her, but my mum was right: I was not ready to be independent with my food.

I certainly started strong, but after a couple of weeks of being the only girl with a snack, I felt the old insecurities creep back in. I started comparing my body to my friends'. Thoughts like 'I should have smaller thighs like her' and 'they don't eat half as much as me; I should stop before I start looking like the chubby one in the group' fed my core fear of not being enough. At first, I innocently offered to share my snacks with the others. Later it evolved into so much more. I began to slip back into my anorexia, lose weight, and put my health in jeopardy again.

The Rebellious Act

In a world where we are programmed to compare ourselves to others—from our grades and our income to our weight and our appearance—letting go of comparison takes practice.

The first step, as with many of the rebellious acts in this book, is to pay attention. What are you shoulding on yourself over? Why?

In the case of my skin tone, I had become self-conscious of it even before moving to the U.S. I was walking down the street in England one summer day, and a guy actually took the time to stop, roll down his window, and holler at me to 'go get a tan'. That stayed with me for years, but I didn't realise how big an effect it had until I started to question my stories.

I'm sure I sound like a broken record by now because awareness really is key to changing anything in life. That's because we operate on autopilot so much of the time and only realise what's happening when it's too late, and we are already down the rabbit hole of judgement, shame, guilt, and comparison.

Your inner mean girl is also very much like a toddler. If you ignore her, she'll get louder. Acknowledging her may seem counterintuitive, but this does not give her more power. In fact, it gives you the power to speak up for yourself. If you hear her in your head, going on about how you're not good enough, simply say, 'I hear you, but I'm not interested in talking right now'.

After recognising what's going on, the next step is to implement self-compassion. If you need to refresh your memory, go back to this rebellious act in chapter 6—words don't do justice in describing how important it is for reclaiming unconditional love for your body.

When you realise you're comparing yourself to others, the kindest thing you can do is recognise that you can't possibly compare yourself to anyone else on the planet because we're all unique. It's literally like comparing the sun and the moon. They both shine but in completely different ways. When you get into comparison, you dim your own unique light. Would you let your inner child dim her light as everyone else shines? Or would you nurture her so she can glow?

As we know, reframing things is beyond powerful, and this is no different. Seeing comparison in a different way and using a different perspective can be all you need to stop comparison in its tracks and achieve unconditional love for your body.

A powerful tool I absolutely adore for fast-tracking the process of reframing is a gratitude list. Nothing stops the negative mental spiral faster than a bit of gratitude for what we already have.

Our brains tend to have a bias towards looking for the negative as opposed to the positive. This all goes back to survival and keeping us safe. However, unless we are on vacation in the wild, most of us no longer need to worry about being bitten in the butt by a deadly snake or trampled by a herd of rhino. It is okay for us to guide our brains to focus on the good stuff. In fact, it's essential for freeing ourselves from the trap of feeling like we are 'not enough'. We can do this through practicing gratitude.

The beauty of gratitude is that even if you find it hard to appreciate your body, you can still find gratitude in some area of your life, so you can always start there. What you'll find is a domino effect. When you are actively looking for the good stuff around you, you will naturally start finding more positive things about your body also.

The Exercise

Let's test this out. Turn to your journal now and list three things that you are grateful for in your life and then three things you are grateful for regarding your body. This could include what it looks like, what it does for you, or just the fact that it is healthy. Don't overthink here—just write what comes to mind.

For me, I am grateful for the following:

♥ My beautiful home in SoCal that's close to the beach

♥ My loving and supportive parents, partner, and friends

♥ My cute little cat who likes to snuggle up with me when I write

♥ My hands, which I'm using to type this book

♥ My legs for dancing (see chapter 8)

♥ My clear, beautiful, undamaged skin

Make it a daily habit (with the help of a habit tracker) to come back to your list, reread what you have written, and add to it. I like to record my gratitude list on my phone as a voice memo and listen to it in the morning when I wake up, when I go on my walks, and at night before I go to bed.

You can also practice gratitude by simply receiving compliments. Many of us will not take a damn compliment; we're great at giving but receiving does not always come as naturally! We either feel like we must send something back to the other person, deflect or minimise the compliment. However, if you can't take a compliment from others, imagine how challenging you'll find complimenting yourself, practicing gratitude, and having unconditional love for your body.

Rather, I encourage you to get comfortable with receiving a compliment, saying 'thank you', and leaving it at that. Really let the compliment sink in and let yourself feel it. You could even start making a note of compliments you receive and add some of these to your gratitude list.

The Battle

So, you're doing all this fantastic work, writing and listening to your gratitude list daily, and accepting compliments. Then, you open social media. *Bam*—the first thing you see is another woman who immediately sets off the comparison crazies. It can happen instantaneously, hurt deeply, and happen often. In a Huffington Post poll, 60% of social media users reported that it has impacted their self-esteem in a negative way.[19]

I've been there! When I first moved in with Steve and was still in my highly self-conscious phase, I used to get so riled up when I caught a glimpse of his Facebook feed. 'He has so many gorgeous female friends', I thought. It became even worse as I built more connections, and my 'suggested friends' list included these women. Despite receiving compliments myself, I became more and more critical of what I looked like and how I didn't measure up against others.

Alternatively, it's possible you may be comparing your present self to your past self. Whilst working with Vivian on the mirror exercise in chapter 3, I discovered she was comparing photos of herself from the years before her son was born to what she saw in the mirror today. Old photos popping up on her social media news feed set off her inner mean girl, where she would focus on the ways her body had changed and hate on how it currently looked. This was preventing her from developing unconditional love for her body.

If you're ever in a similar situation to Vivian or myself, the best piece of advice I can give you is to unfollow, mute, or press 'delete' ASAP. This is about you protecting your inner peace and nothing more than that. If there is someone or something (such as an old photo) that makes you feel less than, just like you did with the thoughts that made you feel less than, you can dismiss them and move on to people, pictures, and stories that do make you feel strong and empowered.

I've had to do this several times; if the stories of 'not enough' start creeping in, I know what I've got to do. Of course, you still need to be doing all the other work alongside this. However, sometimes letting go is the best thing you can do.

The Summary

Letting go of comparison is a total game changer in the journey of reclaiming your right to unconditional love for your body. It creates an opening for self-acceptance and inner peace. Celebrating your uniqueness and being grateful for your body—what it looks like and how it works—is the key to this. Once you master this, there really is no stopping your inner light from glowing bright.

If you're like most people, you fall back into old patterns within weeks of trying to change a habit, including the habit of gratitude. That's why I'm gifting you an epic habit tracker that I personally use and recommend to all my private clients! Head to www.nutritionbylizzy.com/goodies. No sign up or subscription is required.

RA 12

HAVE A *cheer* SQUAD

If you try to carry your heavy burdens all alone, you will eventually collapse under their weight.

Reclaiming your right to unconditional love for your body is an inside job. It's something only you can do for yourself. That does not, however, imply that you must embark on your journey alone. In reality, having a cheer squad by your side might be your secret weapon in pulling off this ultimate rebellious act.

The Illusion

Our culture attaches a badge of honour to martyrdom in the form of putting ourselves last and working until our eyes bleed, as we discussed in previous chapters. However, there is another element to this: the belief that we must do everything all on our own. It's, without a doubt, the biggest illusion of them all.

I was trapped in this illusion for a very long time. As an only child, I prided myself on my ability to do things on my own. I was perfectly content being alone and didn't need others for amusement. It was something my family praised me for. I was 'so grown up and mature'. How wonderful was I? Well, 'wonderful, independent me' morphed into 'stubborn me' who refused to ask for any help, even when I needed it. I had interpreted the praise to mean that doing it on my own meant 'good' and asking for help meant 'failure'.

As a result, when it came to reclaiming unconditional love for my body, I struggled on my own for years. And, unlike what the movies lead you to believe, there was nothing glamorous or heroic about this struggle.

After rejecting any assistance from my parents and community care team for my eating disorder, that independent streak landed me in the hospital.

This was a godsend for my parents, and they still credit Leigh House for much of my recovery. The hospital listened to what my parents wanted and followed through on it. They were fantastic at what they did and were very supportive.

However, when I was discharged, I reverted back to my old ways, trying to do everything on my own. When I finally plucked up the courage to ask my doctor for help, it was six years later. I was so ashamed of asking for help that I didn't talk to my parents about my health until the results of my bone scan revealed my osteoporosis diagnosis.

I felt totally vulnerable, and it terrified me to finally allow other people to help. I was afraid that others would see me as a failure who couldn't look after herself. I was afraid they would take over my care, just as they did when I was hospitalised, and I would lose all my independence.

I'm not one to dismiss the importance of being independent and taking responsibility for our lives, but once again, it's the intention that counts. You may find yourself in a similar situation to mine, where you want to do everything by yourself out of sheer stubbornness.

You might also be afraid of letting others in because you don't like being vulnerable. Perhaps you consider asking for help a sign of failure. All these are negative reasons to go it alone.

Wanting to go it alone implies that you are attempting to carry the full weight of your goals and challenges on your shoulders for the entire journey. This is extremely difficult and exhausting.

If you try to carry your heavy burdens all alone, you will eventually collapse under their weight. On the other hand, if someone you trust is there to guide you and help lighten the load, you have a better chance of succeeding.

Consider it like an endurance race. The professionals never compete alone—they always have a support team on hand. They are the ones who are running the race, but backup is always available should they require a little nourishment (literally or metaphorically). That backup is critical to their success in finishing the race.

If you're sitting there reading this and thinking, 'Well, I'm not a marathon runner', I hear you. Even if you've never played sports, never collaborated with others on a project, never been in a band, or have never been in any type of team situation, you are a human who interacts with other humans every single day. Our very nature necessitates connection. It must take place. The key is whether you choose to embrace this and how you do so.

The Rebellious Act

I mentioned earlier how important connection is in our journey to reclaiming unconditional love for our bodies. If you need a refresher, return to chapter 5.

The easiest way to nurture connection is to form a group of people around you—your cheer squad—who are aware of your goals and want to see you succeed. Those closest to you, such as your partner, parents, and best friend, are among these people.

As I discovered, they are an essential part of any long journey like this. Not only can they provide verbal encouragement and a hug when it's needed the most, but they also understand what you've been through and will be there to celebrate as you progress on your mission to reclaim unconditional love for your body.

You may also live with a partner, parents, or best friend, so it's vital they are aware of your goals, the old patterns you want to break, and the new ones you are forming. This is so they know how they can best support you.

Your loving spouse, for example, may surprise you with a fancy bottle of wine to drink with your Friday night dinner. Really thoughtful, right? Only, your goal is to practice having more love for your body by reducing your alcohol consumption. You go along with it, however, and drink the wine to avoid hurting his feelings whilst thanking him for the beautiful gesture. He does the same thing the following week, completely oblivious to your goals.

If the people closest to you are unaware of or do not understand your goals, they can be huge barriers to achieving unconditional love for your body. On the other hand, they can be amazing assets in your journey when consulted about the changes you're making and may even serve as accountability partners.

Returning to the above example, if you tell your husband about your goals, he may agree to stop buying wine and instead surprise you with flowers. He may also decide to cut back on his alcohol consumption along with you.

Friends and family may be affected by the changes you are making, so having their support and understanding is essential. Your friends, for example, may notice that you no longer want to stay up as late on Saturday nights because you're now taking care of your body by getting enough sleep. If you're the designated driver, they may have to adapt. Knowing your goals, your friends will be able to support you without feeling blindsided.

Another key group to enlist in your cheer squad are your work colleagues. Whilst you may not have as close a relationship with co-workers and are unlikely to share in the same way you would your friends and family, you probably spend at least 40 hours of the week at work. For that reason, you may need to have some support there as well.

Saying 'no' to the cakes that go around the office every Friday, for example, may demonstrate more love for your body. In the interest of diffusing peer pressure, it can be beneficial to mention you are taking care of your health and offer to make an alternative to bring in. Again, you may find that others join you.

Sometimes asking for help from professionals is needed alongside the support you receive from those in your inner circle of friends, family, and work colleagues. Inevitably, there will be speed bumps in your journey of reclaiming unconditional love for your body, and these experts can help you identify ways to overcome them. Nutritionists, personal trainers, and wellness coaches have seen it all before and know how best to deal with any barriers you may face. Their unique expertise will increase the likelihood of you achieving your goals.

Rather than hiring several experts at once, I highly recommend enlisting one expert to work with on a more intensive basis. Whilst it may be tempting to try covering several areas with several different people, sticking to one person helps to avoid confusion and overwhelm on your part. Everyone has their own unique approach, so take the time to find someone with whom you really connect and stick with them.

That isn't to say you can't get advice from other experts by reading books and listening to podcasts. For example, I've recommended several books within these pages that were extremely beneficial to me. As a reminder, these are:

- ♥ *The 5 Love Languages* by Gary Chapman,
- ♥ *The Gifts of Imperfection* by Brené Brown, and
- ♥ *The Diet Fix* by Yoni Freedhoff.

The Exercise

Okay, ladies, this is your final exercise and probably one of the easiest out of all 12 I've given you so far. You have no excuses because it's so simple. Turn to your journal and start writing now!

Make a list of people in your life whom you want to enlist to be on your cheer squad. Think about recruiting your parents, partner, best friend, siblings, grandparents, and work colleagues.

Next, think beyond your inner circle to the type of professionals you might want to work with, such as a nutritionist, personal trainer, or wellness coach. If you know of a specific professional, make note of the person who comes to mind (remember to select only one professional here). For example, you might write my name down if you're looking to dive deeper into the topics covered in this book.

Finally, list any books or podcasts you have come across that you enjoyed in the past and any that you've heard of and want to check out.

Congratulations, you now have your cheer squad!

The Battle

Although I said that this exercise is easy, I encourage you to still be selective when choosing your cheer squad. Choose only those you trust will be supportive and whom you feel aligned with.

In my journey, I made the mistake of asking for support from a community that I didn't know very well. As they were a group of nutritionists who had also recovered from eating disorders, I naively assumed that my background would resonate with them, and so I jumped in to ask for help in spreading the word about this book. I explained my mission was to help as many women as possible develop unconditional love for their bodies. However, it turns out my interpretation of what this entails differed greatly from that group.

Some of my clients want to lose weight as part of their overall journey with me. However, the group accused me of promoting weight loss because of this and went to the extreme of suggesting I didn't care about self-love. Where I expected to find support, I found resistance. This was no big deal. At that point, I recognised a difference in beliefs, chose to wish the group well, and learnt a lesson in selecting my cheer squad.

You may discover there are differences in beliefs between you and others, including your closest friends and family. For example, in identifying your best friend as someone who you want front and centre in your journey, you have a chat with her about your goals and some of the things you're hoping to change. She is overjoyed for you and pledges her full support. The next day, however, she emails you a link to the latest juice cleanse. You can feel yourself becoming frustrated. Although she means well, her interpretation of self-love is different than yours.

This is where being clear and setting boundaries for how you want to be supported comes in handy. It's not your responsibility to persuade your best friend to stop doing her juice cleanse. It is, however, your choice to say, 'no, thank you', and do what is best for you and your body.

Hannah found herself in this position—her friends insisted that a boob job would fix all her body-image issues. After all, it had worked for them, they claimed. However, Hannah didn't want to take the risk of surgery and was sure there was another way. Despite her friends' constant pressure, she worked with me to make the ultimate act of learning to love her natural body unconditionally.

Those who are close to you might not support you at all. For example, in my journey to get this book published, I turned to my family for help. Whilst my parents were enthusiastic, my extended family was not. In the past, that would have caused me to shame myself for asking for help and, in turn, prevent me from being vulnerable and, ultimately, from writing this book. But because I've done a lot of inner work, I could accept their beliefs, keep them separate from my own, and have the self-confidence and trust that I'd be able to do this no matter what.

Indeed, you may find that your initial squad needs some fine-tuning as you enlist them to help in your journey. This may simply involve you changing up your reading list as you discover authors who resonate with you. For me, it was putting my parents and partner in the front row and allowing the rest of my family to observe me from behind, without judgement. And that's the point. It's fine to ask for help; it's also fine for people to say 'no' or to make their own interpretations. I simply keep making the most empowering choices for myself and encourage you to do the same.

The Summary

Although the journey to unconditional love for your body is yours, you don't have to do it on your own. In fact, I'd argue that it's essential you don't do it on your own.

Create a cheer squad with people who you know will support you from the side-lines and share your vision. These people are freaking amazing, so enjoy sharing the process and building deep connections with them.

I personally love working with clients because of the incredible relationships I develop. Many of my clients become long-term friends (and a lot of my long-term friends also become my clients).

I currently work with a small select group clients so that I can fully pour into and witness them totally transform their body confidence, health and energy levels. If you're looking for this personalised, in depth support head to www.nutritionbylizzy.com/about for more information.

THE *pep* TALK

The benefits of being in the Goldilocks zone are massive and
extend beyond simply having the body you desire.

We are all born with the capacity to love our bodies unconditionally. However, our experiences in the world cause us to lose
our sense of self-worth and develop destructive thoughts and
harmful behaviours.

In this book, I have provided you with 12 rebellious acts to
reclaim your right to unconditional love for your body. These
acts are all about letting go of judgement, shame, fear, regret,
and guilt and, instead, empowering yourself to experience joy,
find inner peace, and confidently step into the body you love.

This process involves turning your back on what no longer
serves you and re-establishing balance in your life. As an example, a woman who loves her body unconditionally doesn't
exercise every hour of every day or work herself to exhaustion.

She does not spend her days putting everyone else first or eating junk food for every meal.

Instead, the woman who loves her body unconditionally sits in the middle of extremes, valuing herself and trusting her own judgement. I like to refer to this as operating within your 'Goldilocks zone'.

As I have demonstrated throughout this book, the benefits of being in the Goldilocks zone are massive and extend beyond simply having the body you desire. They affect your time, energy levels, relationships, and bank account.

Indeed, having unconditional love for your body is the greatest gift, but one that can only be given by yourself. It has been an honour to share my personal journey with you and the exercises that have helped me over the years. Now it is your responsibility to take these and put them into practice consistently, with unwavering commitment to yourself. This decision to do so is what shapes a rebel who loves her body unconditionally.

If you're ready to take things to the next level, my self-paced program Reclaim the Rebel Academy is for you. Head to www.nutritionbylizzy.com/rebel to discover how to ditch the diets, silence your inner mean girl and confidently step into the body you love in just 8 weeks.

AFTER *the* REBELLION

My life totally transformed after I fully committed to rebelling against the story that 'I'm not enough' and learnt how to love my body unconditionally. I am now a healthy, fit 31-year-old, Steve and I are married, and I have a thriving coaching business based out of Los Angeles, California.

In my spare time, I cook and bake nutritious food, run for fun, and go on spa days with my best friend. I go to bed when I'm tired, have a habit of daily self-hypnosis and gratitude journaling, and feel comfortable in my own skin.

Don't get me wrong, there are still days where I need to give myself a little more grace, and I don't always 'get it right'. But that's okay: I pick my inner child up, give her a hug, and remind her to go have fun being the rebel she is.

In doing the work myself, I can understand all that my clients, girlfriends, and family members go through and provide a way to support as many women as possible in learning the ultimate act of loving their bodies unconditionally.

I'm living my purpose, and that's the best part. With that, I want to thank you for reading this book and allowing me to serve you.

With love,

Lizzy x

REBEL *journal*

_____

_____

_____

_____

_____

_____

_____

_____

_____

_____

_____

_____

_____

_____

_____

_____

_____

_____

_____

RECLAIM THE REBEL

RECLAIM THE REBEL

RECLAIM THE REBEL

RECLAIM THE REBEL

ACKNOWLEDEGMENTS

I express my deepest gratitude to Julie Cole, Russ Cole, Steve Cangro, Louise Ormerod, Elizabeth Fullbrook, Julie Braden, Sara Drury, Jim Fortin, the Book Launchers team, and all my wonderful clients. Thank you for inspiring me to write this book.

ENDNOTES

1   Jim Fortin, "The Jim Fortin Podcast - E129 - Be Do Have Transformation Series - Part 1 Sneak Peek," www.youtube.com, September 8, 2020, https://www.youtube.com/watch?v=3df1PV6kvv0.

2   Jessica Estrada, "How Your Perception is Your Reality, According to Psychologists," Well+Good, February 7, 2020, https://www.wellandgood.com/perception-is-reality/.

3   Kristine Thomason, "5 Rules for Loving Your Body from Model Ashley Graham," Yahoo! News, January 16, 2016, https://news.yahoo.com/news/5-rules-for-loving-your-body-1343975580008502.html.

4   "Our research," Dove, accessed June 22, 2021, https://www.dove.com/us/en/stories/about-dove/our-research.html.

5   "Body Image & Nutrition: Fast Facts," Teen Health and the Media (Teen Futures Media Network), accessed June 22, 2021, https://depts.washington.edu/thmedia/view.cgi?section=bodyimage&page=fastfacts.

6   Dove Self-Esteem Project, "Girls and Beauty Confidence: The Global Report," *Dove*, 2017, https://www.unilever.com/Images/dove-girls-beauty-confidence-report-infographic_tcm244-511240_en.pdf.

7   "Self-Esteem," The University of Texas at Austin Counseling and Mental Health Center, accessed June 22, 2021, https://cmhc.utexas.edu/selfesteem.html.

8   Elizabeth Venzin, "How Does Low Self-Esteem Negatively Affect You?" Psych Central, March 1, 2014, https://psychcentral.com/blog/how-does-low-self-esteem-negatively-affect-you#1.

9   Gary Chapman, *The 5 Love Languages: The Secret to Love That Lasts* (Chicago, IL: Northfield Publishing, 2015).

10 Brené Brown, *The Gifts of Imperfection: Let Go of Who You Think You're Supposed to Be and Embrace Who You Are* (Center City, MN: Hazelden Publishing, 2010).

11 D. J. Farrell and L. Bower, "Fatal Water Intoxication," *Journal of Clinical Pathology* 56, (September 26, 2003): 803–4, https://www.doi.org/10.1136/jcp.56.10.803-a.

12 Yoni Freedoff, *The Diet Fix: Why Diets Fail and How to Make Yours Work* (New York, NY: Harmony, 2014).

13 Joanne Slavin and Justin Carlson, "Carbohydrates," *Advances in Nutrition* 5, no. 6 (November 3, 2014): 760–61, https://www.doi.org/10.3945/an.114.006163.

14 Francesco P. Cappuccio et al., "Sleep Duration Predicts Cardiovascular Outcomes: A Systematic Review and Meta-Analysis of Prospective Studies," *European Heart Journal* 32, no. 12 (June 2011): 1484–92, https://www.doi.org/10.1093/eurheartj/ehr007.

15 Daniel J. Gottlieb et al., "Association of Sleep Time with Diabetes Mellitus and Impaired Glucose Intolerance," *Archives of Internal Medicine* 165, no. 8 (April 25, 2005): 863–67, https://www.doi.org/10.1001/archinte.165.8.863.

16 Francesco p. Cappuccio et al., "Quantity and Quality of Sleep and Incidence of Type 2 Diabetes: A Systemic Review and Meta-Analysis," *Diabetes Care* 33, no. 2 (February 2010): 414–20, https://www.doi.org/10.2337/dc09-1124.

17 Eric Suni, "Sleep and Overeating," Sleep Foundation, updated November 20, 2020, https://www.sleepfoundation.org/physical-health/sleep-and-overeating.

18 Mark P. Jensen, Tomonori Adachi, and Shahin Hakimian, "Brain Oscillations, Hypnosis, and Hypnotizability," *American Journal of Clinical Hypnosis* 57, no. 3 (January 13, 2015): 230–53, https://www.doi.org/10.1080/00029157.2014.976786.

19 Clarissa Silva, "Social Media's Impact on Self-Esteem," Huffington Post, updated February 22, 2017, https://www.huffpost.com/entry/social-medias-impact-on-self-esteem_b_58ade038e4b0d818c4f0a4e4.

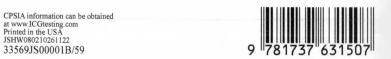